Combat Veterans:

Bringing It Home

A Survival Guide for
Combat Veterans and their Loved Ones

Bill DeWitt, MA, MFT
Viet Nam, 1967-68

Dear Ben,

This will most likely help explain my journey back from Viet Nam.

If my guy Robbie ever considern putting on a uniform, please tie him down until he reads this cover to cover.

Hugs
YOUR BRO

There are some things that cannot be learned quickly, and time, which is all we have, must be paid heavily for their acquiring.
They are the very simplest things, and because it takes a man's life to know them, they are very costly to him and the only heritage he has to leave.

Ernst Hemingway

Combat Veterans

Acknowledgments

The foundation of this book is built upon the collective work of an amazing group of writers, psychotherapists and historians.

I wish to thank Stephen Ambrose, Paul Fussell, Richard Holmes, Jon Krakauer and Gerald Linderman for their insight into the experience of the individual in combat. David Hackworth, Ronald Glasser, Robert Mason, Don Malarkey, William Manchester, Clint Van Winkle and Paul Reickhoff carry that dialogue even further with rich, first-person accounts of combat survival. We have John Keegan, Bruce Catton, John Dower, Shelby Foote and Max Hastings to thank for creating a broader context through which to view the larger historical patterns.

Through the work of Judith Herman, Joseph LeDoux and Amanda Ripley, I have gained a clearer view of the intricacies of the individual process. I am grateful for the insights into marriage and family that I have garnered over the years from John Gottman, Virginia Satir, Chuck Holt, Meri Shadley, Carl Whittaker, Mary Pipher, Christiane Northrup and many others too numerous to mention. As well, the writings of Ursula Le Guin, Barbara Kingsolver, Louis De Bernieres, Lewis Thomas and Tom Robbins have all left their indelible mark upon me.

I am deeply appreciative of the feedback, affirmation and unfailing support of Charlotte and Sophie DeWitt, without which this book would not have been possible.

The following folks have been instrumental in making this book a reality: John Dorf, Judy Holt, Bruce Mayhall, Cornelius Caporani, Michael Fowle, Sue Collins, Susan Trabucco, Keith Albers, Tim Wilson and Bernie Wood.

To Peter Gearin goes a special thank you for his creative and masterful work in layout and cover design.

Combat Veterans

I also want thank my comrades of Company B, 1/52nd Infantry for their courage and sacrifice in combat. Among them, there are two that deserve special acknowledgment: Capt. Gary Goldman for his leadership, determination and self-sacrifice in buffering us from the insanity of a deeply flawed command structure; and secondly, Sgt. Leonard "Dutch" Dutcher, who took point when he didn't have to.

Dutch died in June, 1968, Killed in Action.

Table of Contents

Introduction   9

A User's Guide   11

Part I: What They Didn't Tell You   13
Command Incompetence: The War Lovers; The Distant
Commanders; Fighting the Last War;
    Butchers and Boneheads
- The Obscene Brutality of War: The Clean Machine;
  The Large Scale; The Bizarre Small Scale; As Culture;
  POWs

Part II: The Spiral   51
- The foundation of the Spiral; The Amygdala.
- Survivorship: Denial, Deliberation, Decision.
- Combat: Denial to Deliberation.
- Battlewise: The Spiral of Combat
- The Spiral I: Numbing/Toughening/A Shrinking
  Universe
- The Spiral II: Counterpoints, Combat Distress, Fatalism
- The Spiral III: Exhaustion

Part III: Bringing It Home   91
- Integrating Two Worlds: Stanger in a Strange Land;
  Vets and Therapy
- A Tool Kit: John Gottman/Marriage;
  The Alarm Reaction; Flooding; The Four Horsemen;
- Looking at Family: Rigid Roles; Triangles;
  Anticipating; Rites of Passage; Reflexive Payback;
  Fragility of Life; Suicide
- The Authority Bully

- Healing: Disconnection; Small Scale; Large Scale
- The Damaged Self

Part IV: The Nature of War   **143**
- Endless Wars; High Purpose, Noble Goals
- War Evolves: The Evolution of War
- Patterns Emerge
- War: A Power unto Itself

Bibliography   **157**

Introduction

This book is written specifically for Combat Veterans and their loved ones by one of their own.

Combat Vets returning from Iraq/Afghanistan, as well as those who have come home from previous wars, will find precious insights in these pages that honestly and accurately reflect their experience. They will also find a clear and helpful exploration of that huge leap every Combat Vet must make as they leave the world of War and try to complete the journey home.

This book offers Combat Vets a perspective into the universality of the human experience of War. Their Loved Ones will be given a glimpse into a world far different than their own. It is a glimpse that will help to engender understanding.

This book is both broad and narrow in scope.

We will begin by taking a direct look at the dark underbelly of combat. We'll look at the nasty stuff that normally gets pushed aside, kept politely out of sight. The process is painful and dark but the truth of it needs to be hauled out into the light. Again, it will help Loved Ones to begin to understand.

As we narrow our view, we will look at the detailed experiences of many Combat Veterans, as described in their own words, so as to get it exactly right. We will closely track the journey of several extraordinary Vets as they share their story with the author while working in psychotherapy to reduce residual combat pain.

We will also explore the latest research that reveals new insights about stress, the brain, trauma and recovery. We'll explore the concept of

'Survivorship', how it applies to **the Spiral** of combat and what it all means to Combat Vets down the road.

We will weave these threads together to create both insight and a practical helping hand in the process of **Bringing It Home**.

Finally, we will examine the evolution of War over the centuries. As a guide, we will use insights carefully selected from the writings of a small group of gifted historians. These are men and women who have dedicated their life's work to understanding the complexity of War.

Lastly, this is the book I wish I could have had at my side when I was puked out of the hell of the Viet Nam War, emotionally, physically and spiritually exhausted.

A User's Guide

Please use this book to serve your specific needs.

It has been designed to be a useful tool, not an academic exercise.
It has been written in such a way as to build a step-wise map of the
complex world of combat.

However, this broad approach may not suit your needs.

If you, as a Combat Veteran, are struggling to come to grips with the
huge gap between the noble promises of the recruiting machine and the
bitter reality of combat, then **Part I: What They Didn't Tell You** will
be a good place to start.

Or, you may choose, instead, to immediately focus on a different,
'Part' that is more immediately important to you (without working
through another 'Part' that is of less importance to you).

For example: if your primary concern is to gain a specific
understanding of how the stress of combat impacts the individual, you
may want to move directly to **Part II: the Spiral**.

As a Loved One, you may be most concerned with the process of
coming home, of reintegration with the family. Then you (and your
Vet) may choose to begin by exploring **Part III: Bringing It Home.**

Each one of the four Parts is interlaced with valuable ideas and
references, which point to areas of further exploration.

For example: **Part IV: The Nature of War** presents an overview of
the evolution of war. It creates a context within which to better
understand the current wars in Iraq/Afghanistan. It is engaging stuff

[11]

that offers a broad overview of war that may be insightful and healing to any Combat Vet struggling to come to terms with their experience.

So, use this book as a tool to focus on your primary concerns without getting sidetracked.

Also, a quick word about what you won't find here:
You will not find information specific to the clinical criteria for diagnosis of PTSD nor its clinical treatment.

Similarly, you will not find information about accessing Veteran's benefits or dealing with the VA. If either of these areas are your main concern, there are many other resources available that will be much more useful than this book.

Part I: What They Didn't Tell You

For many Combat Veterans, there is a huge disconnect between the expectations they carry into combat and their personal experience of war. No matter how motivated or well trained, most Vets find the realities of combat to be laced with brutal truths that can often be staggering. We will explore some of these truths that won't be highlighted in the recruiting ads running during the halftime show of the Super Bowl. They are truths that pervade the world of war and become a stark reality for most Combat Veterans only after being buried up to the neck in their ugliness.

What they didn't tell us:

Command Incompetence

Saving Kuwait City

Randy had his act pretty together. As we began our first psychotherapy session in my office, it quickly became clear that what Randy mainly needed was some feedback. He wasn't dealing very well with his hot 'n sexy, sometimes-a-lunatic live-in babe (who he both loved and hated). Filling in some background, he talked about his four-year career in the Marine Corps that had just recently ended.

He had a love/hate relationship with the Corps as well.

Randy definitely loved the challenges he had faced as a Marine, pushing himself both mentally and physically. He quickly picked up stripes, finally leading his squad, mounted on their own amphibious troop carrier, northward into the desert during Operation Desert Storm. They were on their way to liberate Kuwait. His battalion took great pride in the fact that it had been chosen to be the cutting edge, the very tip of the spear. They would lead the 2nd Marine Division through the mass of Iraqi armor and artillery standing

[13]

between them and Kuwait City. It was exciting stuff, for a while at least.

"You know, it wasn't so bad, at first. We caught the Iraqis totally off guard. Didn't run into much resistance until we got up around Khaffi, up on the Saudi border. That was a little hairy. But the Cobras came up and did their thing. So, up to that point, we hadn't taken any casualties."

"The problem was, we had this major up at battalion ops who was just a relentless son-of-a bitch. He told everybody that he was going to personally liberate Kuwait City and he didn't give a screamin' shit what it would take to do it."

Randy clenched and unclenched his fists a couple of times while I quietly listened and waited.

"Pretty soon we couldn't get any fire support because we'd outrun our artillery. Then we had a hard time getting any air support because of shitty commo links. It was so bad sometimes; we couldn't even raise battalion on the radio net."

He clenched and unclenched again.

"Finally, we had to stop 'cause our logistics train couldn't catch up. We were totally running out of fuel and water. It just sucked that we were scattered all over hell and back, but what are you goin' to do? We just decided to button up for the night, hoping things'd get straightened out in the morning.

"So, we're all sacked out, catching some zzz's. Then, a couple of hours later, we hear this knocking on the door of the track. Scared the shit outta' us, right?!! So, we scramble up top and there, outside, gathered all around our carrier, is like at least a hundred Iraqis, trying to surrender.

"Good thing they weren't into fightin' 'cause our shit was totally exposed. Just 'cause this major asshole wanted to get his medals and his promotion."

Randy shook his head in disgust.

"And, you know, sometimes it just doesn't work out for jerks like that…"

"He wasn't first into Kuwait City?" I asked.

Randy smiled.

"Not quite! We got all the way up to the seventh ring road, just outside the City. Word came down from division that we needed to stand aside. They wanted the Saudis and Kuwaitis, back down the road somewhere, to come up and liberate the place. Show the Arab flag and all that happy horseshit…"

"Pissed the major off, yeah?"

Randy smiled briefly.

"Sure did! But what's important is, I realized right there I had to get the hell outta' the Corps as soon as I could."

Randy wasn't smiling anymore.

"You know, you suddenly figure out you got some son-of-a-bitch in charge of your life who, underneath all the rah-rah heroes stuff, doesn't really give a crap if you live or die. All he really gives a shit about is getting his ticket punched. It's a real wake up…"

The Same Old Dance

Some of us who have survived combat were blessed with a commander who made the survival of their troops a top priority; commanders who knew how to take care of their troops without compromising the success of the mission.

Others of us have had firsthand experience with the tragic truth behind Randy's story.

As an infantry company commander in Vietnam, I was forced to fight a bitter and endless battle with a fool; a battalion S-3 (also a major) who insisted, time after time that I send my men into danger unnecessarily. He refused to listen to reason or take into account my on-the-ground observations. He issued his orders from the safety of a sandbagged TOC (Tactical Operations Center) command bunker, six klicks to the rear.

To this day, I hold him solely responsible for the death of my colleague, (a fellow company commander, a West Point graduate finishing his 2nd tour in Vietnam) who would have put his whole career in jeopardy if he had refused to comply with the major's last insane command.

Instead he obeyed and died, along with too many of his troops.

[15]

It's the same old dance that has happened over and over again, over the years, over the decades, even over the centuries.

It is a pattern that is worth looking at in detail.

Command Incompetence: The War Lovers

George Armstrong Custer Dashes to Glory

Custer lost his life and his command at the hands of the Sioux in 1876 because of characteristics he had displayed time and again in the Civil War. His undoubted audacity and courage were offset by a criminal lack of good judgment, a refusal to take the time to gather intelligence about the enemy, an insistence on attacking at the earliest possible opportunity, a petty jealousy towards his fellow officers, a monumental ambition, and a total disregard for the lives of his men. (Ambrose, Americans 48)

This is powerfully critical language ("…a criminal lack of good judgment…") coming from Stephen Ambrose, a remarkable historian and a steadfast American patriot. But he has the courage to speak the truth. Other famous military icons don't show up so well in the light of day, either.

George S. Patton: Old Blood and Guts

While there are few who would argue with the fact of his brilliant battlefield successes, there are many who believed Patton to also be a world class "martinet" (a petty dictator) who loved the dramatic stage war offered him and played it for all its worth:

General Patton had more than a bit of the chicken shit in him. He was notorious for being a martinet about dress and spit-and-polish in the Third Army. He ordered-and sometimes may have gotten- frontline infantry to wear ties and shave everyday…Patton's spit-and-polish obsession sometimes cost

[16]

dearly. It not only had nothing to do with the winning of the war, it hurt the war effort. (Ambrose, Citizen 335)

Like Custer, Patton is celebrated today as a brave and noble warrior. Like Custer, Patton seemed to have an actor's sense of the role that he and his fellow commanders must play to perform their part to the hilt.

Paul Fussell, himself an infantry officer in WWII Europe, wrote (after the war) about Patton's mandate to his commanders that they make "appearances" at the front. The further forward the appearance was made, the better, Patton argued; it seemed especially effective with the troops if the commander was seen to be in the presence of danger. Fussell elaborates further:

> As Patton's words appear and effect suggest, he is a master of the difference between external theater and internal actuality. One of his most brilliant suggestions to high officers working on the morale of their troops is never to be seen going to the rear. In visiting the line, go up in a jeep for all to see, but coming back, fly. (Fussell, Wartime 152)

It is interesting that the nickname, "Old Blood and Guts" grew out of a grumbled response one of his infantrymen gave to a question from a reporter: "Yeah, our blood and his guts."

Most telling of all was the confrontation between Patton and his immediate subordinate, Omar Bradley, during the Allied race across Sicily in 1943. Patton was caught up in a battle of egos with General Montgomery, the commander of the British ground forces. Like Patton, Montgomery was pushing his troops hard, demanding that they take the town of Messina before Patton and the Americans could arrive. Bradley repeatedly argued with Patton about the risks that Patton was taking with the lives of his men in the point units. They were taking unnecessary casualties over and over again, simply because Patton was determined to beat Montgomery to

Messina: "There's a big difference between us, George." said General Bradley. "I do this job because I've been trained to do it. You do it because you love it." (D'este 978)

Different war, same old dance.

Band of Brothers Redux

Having fought their way from Normandy through Belgium and Bastogne, to the western border of Germany, some of the troopers of Easy Company, of the 101st Airborne *Band of Brothers*, began to hope that they just might live to see VE Day. On one cold, wintery night in February, 1945, twelve of them were ordered to paddle across a small river, creep into German-held positions and grab prisoners for interrogation. They succeeded, capturing two Germans, making it back across the river at the cost of one friendly KIA. They were hugely relieved to have it behind them.

The following day, however, their regimental commander, Col. Sink, proudly spread the word of his men's accomplishment up and down the chain of command. He was so enormously pleased with his newly-found bragging rights that he figured it would be a grand idea to send out another patrol, again that very same night. It didn't seem to concern him that the Germans would be on a heightened state of alert and things would be a lot tougher the second time around.

Luckily for the troops, Maj. Winters, the 2nd Battalion commander, had been their company commander until his recent promotion. Winters knew firsthand what the weary Vets of Easy Company had been through. Fortunately for them, he was the kind of officer who was unwilling to risk lives unnecessarily. Even so, they were surprised that evening as they sullenly gathered together to begin to prepare for another confrontation with death:

Col. Sink and a couple of staff officers came to 2nd Battalion CP to observe. They had a bottle of whiskey with them. Winters said he was going down to the river bank to supervise the patrol. When he got to the outpost, he told the men to just stay still. With the whiskey working on him, Sink would soon be ready for bed. The patrol could report in the morning that it had gotten across the river and into German lines but had been unable to get a live prisoner. (Ambrose, Band 234)

The same old dance.

Viet Nam Redo

While stationed as a doctor at a US evacuation hospital in Japan in 1968, Ronald Glasser listened closely to the wounded troopers in his care, all of whom were medical evacuees from Viet Nam. He recorded these comments, made by a veteran of the 101st Airborne, a severely wounded patient of his in the Orthopedic Ward: "After six months they promoted our colonel and sent him to Washington. It's not that he's a liar or a bad guy. It's just that he loves this shit. If they listen to him, they're fucken' crazy." (Glasser 179)

Different war, same old dance.

Command Incompetence: The Distant Commander

As technological advances in communication found their way onto the battlefield (telegraph, telephone, wireless radio, email) commanders found themselves further and further physically removed from the battle. The resulting disconnect often resulted in catastrophic losses for the frontline soldier. Occasionally, a courageous commander at the front had the moral strength to countermand orders from the rear that would, if executed, have resulted in disaster for his troops.

A General of Courage: WWI

An example of moral clarity facing off command incompetence; from the trenches of WWI:

Major-General Pilcher, commanding the 17th Division in the summer of 1916, was faced with a similar conflict

[19]

between duty to his superiors and loyalty to his subordinates when ordered to carry out an attack on Mametz Wood. He considered asking to be relieved of his command, but eventually decided to carry on, because a new commander might have got even more men killed. But he did not attack according to plan, and paid the price of disobedience.

"If I had obeyed the corps order more literally,' he wrote, "I should have lost another two or three thousand men and achieved no more. I was, as you know, accused of want of push, and consequently sent home. It is very easy to sit a few miles in the rear, and get the credit for allowing men to be killed in an undertaking foredoomed to failure, but the part did not appeal to me and my protests against these useless attacks were not well received." (Holmes 320)

Many other commanders didn't possess Pilcher's moral clarity. In the absence of such courage, tragedy often blossoms for the common soldier.

A Hopeless Tragedy: The Civil War

In the waning days of the Civil War, Union forces closed in on a section of Confederate trenches just outside of Petersburg, Virginia, that had been accidentally left unoccupied by southern forces. The Union commander, Gen. Meade, is described by Bruce Catton:

....(Meade) was in a foul temper, which kept growing worse and he emitted a furious stream of orders..."I sent an order to each corps commander to attack at all hazards"....

Late in the afternoon, the attacks were finally made. It was too late, by now, for Lee's veterans were in the trenches at last and the eight-to-one odds had vanished forever; this was Cold Harbor all over again, with its cruel demonstration that trench lines properly manned could not be taken by storm. The chance (for success) had gone, and an attack now could result in nothing but destruction for the attackers.

[20]

The soldiers knew this, even if their generals did not. In mid-afternoon Gen. Birney (one of Meade's corps commanders) massed his troops for a final attack as ordered. His principal column was formed in four lines, with veteran troops in the first two lines and oversized heavy artillery regiments, untried but full of enthusiasm, in the last two.

The men were lying down when the order to charge the Rebel works came in, and as the officers shouted and waved their swords the inexperienced artillerists sprang to their feet while the veterans ahead of them continued to lie prone. The veterans looked back, saw the rookies preparing to charge, and called out: "Lie down, you damn fools, you can't take them forts!"

One of the artillery regiments, the 1st Massachusetts Heavies, accepted this advice, lay down again, and made no charge. The other one, the 1st Maine, valiantly stayed on its feet, ran forward through the rows of prostrate men, and made for the Confederate line. It was a hopeless try. The Confederate gun pits had been built low and the black muzzles of the guns that peered evilly out of the embrasures were no more than a foot or two above the ground, and when they fired the canister came in just off the grass so that nobody could escape. The whole slope was burned with fire, and in a few minutes more than 600 of the 900 men in the regiment had been shot down, the ground was covered with mangled bodies, and the survivors were running for the rear. (Catton 197-198)

A General of Courage: The Civil War

In stark contrast, Catton describes one of the "great days" had by Union General Governor Warren, also a subordinate to General Meade:

> ...at Mine Run, in December, half of the Union army had been given to him for a mighty assault that was to destroy the Rebel army and make General Warren a national hero. At

[21]

the last minute, General Warren had discovered that the Confederate line was far stronger than supposed: so strong, indeed, that the attack could not possibly succeed and would be no better than a second Fredericksburg. With no time to refer to the army commander, he had to have the moral stamina to call things off. Let Meade's wrath descend entirely on himself and take whatever rap might be coming. (Catton 51-52)

Tragedy on a 'Delightful Day': WWI

British historian John Keegan describes, in great detail, the activities of the WWI British generals, far in the rear, on the opening day of the Battle of the Somme. Just over the horizon from them, masses of British infantry were being slaughtered in the course of obeying the proscribed general orders. As the generals dallied, the tragedy played itself out, unseen, on the distant horizon:

> Throughout the morning and afternoon,…(the British commander) Haig, in his advanced headquarters at the Chateau de Beauquesne, ten miles to the north, attempted to follow the battle from scraps of imprecise information several hours old. (Haig and his fellow commander) could not make real sense of it. Neither, very wisely, ordered any substantive changes of plan. Many of the gunners, whose fire, if properly directed, would have been so effective in saving British lives, also remained, though closer at hand, inactive spectators: "On the whole," wrote Neil Fraser Tyler of a Lancashire Territorial Field Brigade, "we had a very delightful day, with nothing to do except send numerous reports through to Head Quarters and observe the stupendous spectacle before us. There was nothing to do as regards controlling my battery's fire, as the barrage orders had all been prepared beforehand." (Keegan, Book 262-263)

Amazing words to read: "...on the whole, we had a very delightful day"...as their countrymen were literally dying by the tens of thousands.

Stephen Ambrose draws some interesting parallels to the above, as he describes the situation in which the Allies found themselves, as they chased the remnants of the "defeated" German army across France in the fall of 1944:

> ... a British staff officer from General Haig's headquarters visited the Somme battlefield, a week or so after the battle...the attacks had gone forward, through barbed wire, mud, mines, mortar, and machine-gun fire, fallen back with appalling loss, only to be ordered forward again. This had gone on for weeks. And the officer looked out at the sea of mud and was shocked by his own ignorance. He cried out, "My God! Did we really send men to fight in this?"
>
> ... (the current situation) was getting disturbingly close to the British model...headquarters personnel from battalion on up to Corps and Army found themselves good billets and seldom strayed. In general, the American officers handing down the orders to attack and assigning the objective had no idea what it was like at the front. (Ambrose, Citizen 166)

An Avoidable Tragedy: Afghanistan

Sadly, even the use of modern radio and email communication doesn't prevent commanders in the rear from screwing it up for the boots on the ground. In the moments just before the friendly fire incident that took the life of Army Ranger Pat Tillman in Afghanistan, two different layers of the command structure (far to the rear) insisted upon imposing their orders into a situation that was deteriorating rapidly. Lt. David Uthlaut, the platoon commander on the ground, had his hands tied by the conflicting commands from the rear:

> Uthlaut, steamed, e-mailed back his disagreement (with the latest orders) and then radioed it, hoping that the officers would overhear and amend the command. It meant

splitting his firepower, relying on a local, traveling in daylight and arriving in Manah after sundown, too late to begin clearing operations. Why not move at night and arrive there at dawn, especially after sitting in one place for so long that half the countryside knew his platoon's whereabouts? Objection overruled. (Smith 94)

In his biography of Pat Tillman, Jon Krakauer speaks directly to the disconnect felt by Tillman and his fellow Rangers that evening in Afghanistan:

> ...the Rangers on the ground weren't keen to take unnecessary risks simply to meet an arbitrary bureaucratic timeline set by 'fobbits': officers who seldom ventured beyond the security of the forward operating base (the FOB, in military speak), and therefore, from the grunt's perspective, had no clue what it was actually like to fight a war in this unforgiving country. (Krakauer xvii)

The Same Old Dance: Iraq

Paul Rieckhoff gives us a bird's eye view of the yawning gap between the realities faced by his platoon of grunts on the ground vs. the battalion staff, safely ensconced in the sandbagged safety of their TOC (Tactical Operations Center) compound:

> ...the stockpile of weapons, none of it mattered. In an instant, it became clear to me and my men that the TOC All-Stars were men whose primary concern was for themselves, not their men. We had all feared that it was true, but now we were seeing it for sure. The XO and the rest of the Battalion All-Stars thought the war was over. To them, it may have actually seemed that way. They rarely left the compound, slept in air-conditioning and never got shot at. (Reickhoff 124)

Command Incompetence: Fighting the Last War

Old School Admirals and the Honor of the Royal Navy

The following excerpt from O'Connell's *Of Arms and Men* is a jaw-dropping example as to how the top brass in a tradition-bound military structure can collectively become detached from the real world. Catastrophe usually follows and seems, at the time, totally unavoidable. In this case, O'Connell narrows his focus upon the British Royal Navy as it began to prepare itself for the outbreak of WWI:

> In spite of its many advantages, the Royal Navy was an institution flawed at many points. Time and combat would beat through the impressive façade to reveal a system so tied to a particular set of assumptions as to be practically incapable of adjusting itself to reality. Not having fought for a hundred years, it had rusted from within. And this petrification of thought and action found its material representation in the Royal Navy's utter and complete reliance on the gun. If the Germans treated mines and torpedoes as devices with real possibilities, then this was evidence of their foolishness and inexperience in the eyes of the British. Big guns and big ships won wars. (O'Connell 248)

The British admirals were quite in love with their institutional legends and clearly saw themselves as a step above:

> Yet the submarine was simply not a weapon based on confrontation, and herein lay a major reason for its unpopularity. The whole manner of its attack implied skulking, treachery, and deception – qualities warriors traditionally had disdained. British Admiral A.K. Wilson spoke for the entire naval establishment when he described the submarine as "…underhanded, unfair, and damned un-English." (O'Connell 223)

[25]

You may want to re-read that last sentence. Truly an unbelievable statement! When WWI finally broke out in August, 1914, nothing significant happened in the naval war for the first month. Then, one fine morning, a single German submarine found three British armored cruisers completing a "leisurely sweep". Within the hour all three were sunk:

> Almost fourteen hundred men drowned. In terms of casualties, it was the greatest disaster the Royal Navy had suffered in almost three hundred years. But it was more than that, much more.
>
> Somewhere deep in the imagination of the naval establishment, a laughing voodoo priest had just entered the pristine chapel of nautical orthodoxy. And as he polluted icon after icon, it would gradually become clear that this witch doctor who cast no shadow and waved a contract signed in human blood was man's new partner in warfare – technology, come to collect his due. In some weird approximation revenge, the HMS Dreadnaught would ram and sink (the submarine) in March of 1915. But it was only bravado. There were no real counters for the submarine. (O'Connell 249)

As Americans reading such a story, it's rather tempting to imagine posturing, stiff, self-important British admirals with their heads buried in a dark place. But, could it be that there are American commanders cut from the same cloth? Let's see....

Old School Generals: Lost and Confused in Viet Nam

Lt. Col. David Hackworth was a young, up and coming infantry officer when, in 1966, he was assigned to the Pentagon after returning from his first tour in Viet Nam. He was asked by Gen. Harold Johnson, the Army Chief of Staff at the time, to share his views about the war's progress. It would be his first but clearly not his last confrontation with institutional blindness:

"We've had U.S. Army units in Vietnam for eighteen months," I blurted out. "Almost one-third of the Army is committed to that war. But at Fort Benning there is only a handful of field-grade officers with Vietnam experience, and half of these were advisors. They weren't with U.S. units. We're just not putting our best and most recently experienced combat officers into the school system, which is where I believe they belong. We're sending them everywhere else to get their tickets punched, as if their careers took priority over the war. Vietnam is the toughest war we've ever fought, and we're going at it as though we're fighting World War II all over again."

"Now just a minute, Colonel Hackworth," the General bristled. "In terms of enemy and terrain, the fighting in Vietnam is no different for infantry than when we fought in the Philippines after Pearl Harbor."

"Sir," I said, "that statement is about as far from the truth about the future of the war in Vietnam as I have ever heard!" (Hackworth 550)

Hackworth eventually won Johnson's grudging respect, due to his honesty and directness. Soon thereafter he rotated back to Vietnam as an aide to SLA Marshall, the "unofficial" US Army historian. In the months that followed, Hackworth travelled all over Vietnam in his role as 'Slam' Marshall's aide. Both were given a bird's eye view of the overall situation as he and Marshall moved from one divisional headquarters to next, always as honored guests:

The base-camp mentality in Vietnam was an outgrowth of the static days of the Korean War. Back then the Vietnam-era generals had been majors and lieutenant colonels on the outside looking enviously in; no doubt many of them had thought, 'When I'm a general I'll have that, too' and now that they were, they were going to, even if the base camps had even less in place in this war that they had in the last. In Vietnam, a frontless war, the security requirement alone at these base camps was massive. At the 1st Air Cav, an entire brigade --- fully one third of the division --- was engaged solely in protecting the unit's An Khe home. (Hackworth, 556)

His observations speak to the heart of the institutional 'fighting the last war' that marked our effort in Vietnam. His warnings and those of others like him, who choose to speak the truth even if it would eventually destroy their careers, were never heeded.

The colonels and generals Slam and I met on our trip were, in the main, very much entrenched in the can-do (at all costs) bureaucracy that fostered inflated body counts and the like. As such, they seemed truly blind to the crucial shortcomings in the war effort. It was a bad situation only exacerbated by the obscene luxury available to many at base camps like the 1st Air Cav's and the 1st Division's. Vietnam was as complicated a conflict as the U.S. had ever known, yet the longer many of these generals stayed, the less they understood the war or even tried to, so caught up were they with the finer things in life available in a war zone. I found it interesting that these guys, many of whom had learned little in their last combat commands in the 'sitzkrieg' days of the Korean War, still managed to take the worst of the lessons Korea offered and make them the standard for Vietnam. (Hackworth 573)

Command Incompetence: Butchers and Boneheads

A Butcher's Day at Gettysburg

On a bad day, even the most generally competent and beloved of commanders can make horrible errors of judgment. The results are predictable: death and suffering for those under their command.

This was the case with Robert E. Lee, commanding the Confederate army at the Battle of Gettysburg in July, 1864.

On the third and last day of the battle, the Union infantry had established themselves in a formidable defensive position along the base of Cemetery Ridge. Supporting them where numerous Union artillery batteries, strategically arrayed along the ridge to their immediate rear. The Confederates forces were positioned opposite, along Seminary Ridge, which lay to the west, across three-quarters of a mile of open farmland.

Gen. Lee had somehow made up his mind the evening before that the Union position could and must be taken by frontal assault. He was determined to follow that course of action even if it defied all logic and reason.

Gen. James Longstreet, Lee's trusted second-in-command, repeatedly tried to persuade Lee to change his mind. In the hours leading up to the attack, Longstreet argued that by simply maneuvering around the Union left flank, the Confederates could impose themselves between their enemy and the Union capital, Washington, DC. It would create a situation that could not be tolerated by Meade, the Union commander. Meade's forced choice at that point would be either to attack the Confederates in their new defensive positions or to passively watch while the Confederates attacked Washington at their leisure. Either outcome, Longstreet passionately argued, would result in a resounding Confederate victory.

Lee's response was simple, rigid and mindless:

> "No," Lee said. "I am going to take them where they are on Cemetery Ridge. I want you to take Pickett's division and make the attack."
>
> "That will give me 15,000 men," Longstreet replied. "I have been a soldier all my life, in pretty much all kinds of skirmishes. I think I can safely say there never was a body of 15,000 men who could make that attack successfully." (Davis 236)

Lee flatly refused to reconsider his decision. Reflecting back across the distance of a century, the noted Civil War historian, Shelby Foote, reduced this complex turning point in American history to its essential simplicity: "Bobby Lee had his blood up."

Gen. Longstreet finally withdrew from the futility of the argument, retreating into a deep, depressed silence. He knew full well what lay just ahead, in the bloodbath that is today known as 'Pickett's Charge'.

He was not alone.

Lewis Armistead and Dick Garnett, Confederate generals and close personal friends, shared a quiet moment just before they led their men into the attack. They sat together gazing out across the shimmering expanse awaiting them in the hot July sun. A witness recorded their exchange for posterity:

> Both men were experienced soldiers, and both knew at a glance the ordeal they and their brigades would be exposed to when the signal came for them to advance. Finally, Garnett broke the silence: "This is a desperate thing to attempt," he said. Armistead agreed. "It is," he replied. "But the issue is with the Almighty, and we must leave it in his hands. "(Foote 534)

They did "leave it in his hands" and marched to their own deaths within the hour. Of the 11,000 Confederates who participated in Pickett's Charge, more than 5000 were either killed or captured. Those who survived were scarred and demoralized, their fighting spirit largely broken.

Immediately afterward, Lee declared the fault was entirely his alone. His words were small solace for the Confederate dead carpeting the blood-soaked fields.

For the two previous, bitter years of war the Confederate army had clung to an absolute faith in eventual victory. As a consequence of one rigid, bone-headed decision that faith was drained away, never to return.

A Bonehead Winter in Korea

By early November, 1950, American forces were being pushed further and further north, up into North Korea by their commanders. Higher command was determined to reach the Yalu River (which

[30]

marked the boundary with Communist China) before the onset of winter.

The most ambitious of all of these commanders was Maj. Gen. Edward Almond, a protégée of Gen. Douglas MacArthur. Almond relentlessly pushed the advance of X Corps northward, toward the frozen Chosen Reservoir on Korean's east coast. To many of the officers who worked closely with him, Almond personified a witch's brew of traits that would eventually spell disaster for those under his command.

He was arrogant with a fierce temper. He was totally blind to his own shortcomings. And to cap it off, he was protected by an all-powerful sponsor (MacArthur) and had a consuming lust for glory. One of his staff officers described him this way: "He could not visualize himself being wrong. He was almost as bad as MacArthur in this. Once he made up his mind that something was so, he was just not listening anymore." (Hastings, Korea 160)

Fortunately for the grunts of the 1st Marine Division they had, in the person of their division commander, Gen. O.P. Smith, the mirror opposite of Almond.

Thorough, purposeful and thoughtful, Smith demanded that his Marines be allowed to maintain an adequate supply line as they moved northward from the coast. He created reserve depots of ammunition and supplies at critical points along the Marine line of advance. And, most importantly, he insisted that a 75 mile-long escape route be kept open behind his Marines, as they slowly fought their way up a narrow, icy gravel road. Smith refused to ignore the unknowns: the advent of what would become a horrific Korean winter and the possibility of intervention by the massive Chinese army.

Almond, Smith's immediate commander, was furious with the Marine general. Almond believed that Smith's tardiness was simply a result of an over-cautious pig-headedness. Even after Chinese units began to attack, Almond dismissed their importance. His orders to one of his army commanders were emphatic: "We're still attacking and we're going all the way to the Yalu. Don't let a bunch of Chinese laundrymen stop you." (Hastings, Korea 154)

The two generals were barely speaking to each other by the last week of November, 1950. Suddenly, 100,000 Chinese swarmed southward in the attack, overwhelming the most advanced American units without pause. Initially, Almond refused to acknowledge the urgency of the situation. Then, in a sudden reversal, his limitless ambition turned into barely controlled panic. It dawned upon him that he might be held responsible for a staggering, utterly humiliating American defeat. Searching for any quick way out, Almond suggested that Smith's Marines abandon all their equipment to speed up their withdrawal over the narrow, ice-covered roads; roads which were often attacked from both sides by masses of Chinese infantry.

Smith would have none of it. He knew his men's very survival depended upon a purposeful, orderly withdrawal. His response to Almond was blunt and barely covered his simmering rage: "I'm not going to do that. This is the equipment we fight with." After Almond left Smith's HQ, Smith turned to his staff officer: "This guy is a maniac. He's nuts. I can't believe he's saying these things." (Hastings, Korea 157)

Most competent historians would agree with Smith's assessment of Almond. Smith, on the other hand, was the guy to turn to when all hell broke loose. He boosted Marine morale sky high when he told reporters on Dec. 4th: "Gentlemen, we are not retreating. We are merely advancing in another direction."

The troops got the word. They had a commander they could trust, not a bonehead who would steer them into disaster. They began to believe they could pull off one of the most impossible tactical withdraws in military history… and did.

A Distant Cowboy Plays Bonehead

In July, 2003, George W. Bush, in his role as Commander in Chief, delivered a remarkable speech in which he stared into the camera with steely eyes and welcomed the blossoming insurgency in Iraq to challenge his manhood: "There are some who feel like the conditions are such that they can attack us there (in Iraq). My answer is, bring 'em on."

For the troops on the ground, this casual invitation to violence had real life consequences. Lt. Paul Rieckhoff, serving in Iraq as an infantry platoon leader at the time, had this reaction:

> *Bring 'em on?* What the hell was he thinking? My soldiers and I were searching for car bombs...scanning rooftops for snipers, and our president was in Washington taunting our enemies and encouraging them to attack us. Who the hell did he think he was? He had finally taken the cowboy act too far. Iraq was not a movie and he was not Clint Eastwood. The armchair bravado and arrogance of our commander in chief affected our lives directly and immediately....Iraq was in a very fragile state and we needed our president to be a statesman, not a bully. (Rieckhoff 158)

The Obscene Brutality of War

War: The Clean Machine

Paul Fussell survived his service in WWII Europe as an infantry combat officer to return home and earn a Ph.D. from Harvard. He eventually became a professor of English Literature at the University of Pennsylvania. He is one of the very few academics in the field who can write about War, based upon intimate knowledge and personal experience. His cleared-eyed honesty cuts through a lot of 'official bullshit'. In his book *Wartime* he sets the stage for us:

> In the popular and genteel iconography of war during the bourgeois age, all the way from eighteen- and nineteenth-century history paintings to twentieth-century photographs, the bodies of the dead, if inert, are intact. Bloody, sometimes, sprawled in awkward positions, but except for the absence of life, plausible and acceptable simulacra of the people they once were. But there is a contrary and much more 'realistic' convention represented in, say, the Bayeux Tapestry, where the ornamental border displays numerous severed heads and

limbs. That convention is honored likewise in Renaissance awareness of what happens to the body in battle.

In Shakespeare's Henry V, the soldier Michael Williams assumes the traditional understanding when he observes: "But if the cause be not good, the King himself hath a heavy reckoning to make when all those legs and arms and heads, chopp'd off in a battle, shall join together at the latter day and cry all 'We died at such a place' --- some swearing, some crying for a surgeon, some upon their wives left poor behind them, some upon the debts they owe, some upon their children rawly felt." (268-269)

What Fussell is saying is this: somewhere back three hundred years ago or so, the old images associated with War got cleaned up.

A whole new set of images were created and delivered to the public. These newly popular ideals depicted the adventure of War as epic, admirable and heroic. Totally absent from this new view were torn body parts, crushed skulls, wanton destruction or smashed internal organs, leaking their stench out into the environment. In essence, the brutal, ugly truth was now shunted aside. All the old horrors were to be hidden away. War was to become evermore grand and noble in the popular imagination.

Let's expose this fraud with a simple survey of real events that have happened to real people.

Brutality: The Large Scale

The Bloody Falaise Pocket

In the summer of 1944, the Allies were bursting out of their beachhead in Normandy, encircling major German units from both the north and the south. Hitler demanded that the German army attack and fight to the death, instead of withdrawing to a better defensive position. By obeying his senseless orders the Germans found themselves becoming trapped in a rapidly closing pocket near the French village of Falaise. As their frontline crumbled, a panicked flight eastward, toward relative safety, began to gain momentum. The Americans had complete air superiority and could attack relentlessly. Stephen Ambrose records the Germans' agony in detail:

> For sheer ghastliness in World War II, nothing exceeded the experience of the Germans caught in the Falaise gap. Feelings of helplessness waved over them. They were in a state of total fear day and night. They seldom slept. They dodged from bomb crater to bomb crater. "It was complete chaos," Pvt. Herbert Meier remembered. "That's when I thought, 'This is the end of the world'.
>
> All this time the 1,000-pound bombs, the 500-pound bombs, the rockets, the 105s and the 155s, the 75s on the Shermans, the mortars, and the .50 –caliber machine-gun fire came down on the Germans. Along the roads and in the fields, dead cows, horses, and soldiers swelled in the hot August sun, their mouths agape, filled with flies. Maggots crawled through their wounds. Tanks drove over men in the way – dead or alive. Human and animal intestines made the roads slippery. Maj. William Falvey of the 90th Division recalled seeking 'six horses hitched to a large artillery gun. Four horses were dead and two were still alive. The driver was dead but still had the reins in his hands.' Those few men, German or American, who had not thrown away their gas masks, had them on, to the envy of all the others. The stench was such that even the pilots in the Piper Cubs threw up. (Ambrose, Citizen 103)

Carnage on Okinawa

Within a few months time a similar kind of horror was being replicated on the other side of the world. The US Marines were fighting a grim battle of attrition against Japanese soldiers defending the island of Okinawa. Again, Paul Fussell, *Wartime,* sets the stage for the words of E.B. Sledge, a young Marine who survived that battle:

> But for Sledge, the worst of all was a week-long stay in rain-soaked foxholes on a muddy ridge facing the Japanese, a site strewn with decomposing corpses turning various colors,

nauseating with the stench of death, "an environment so degrading I believed we had been flung into hell's own cesspool." (253).

Because there were no latrines and because there was no moving in daylight, the men relieved themselves in their holes and flung the excrement out into the already foul mud. It was a latter-day Verdun, the Marine occupation of that ridge, where the artillery shelling uncovered scores of half-buried Marine and Japanese bodies, making the position "a stinking compost pile."

"If a Marine slipped and slid down the back slope of the muddy ridge, he was apt to reach the bottom vomiting. I saw more than one man lose his footing and slip and slide all the way to the bottom only to stand up horror-stricken as he watched in disbelief while fat maggots tumbled out of his muddy dungaree pockets, cartridge belt, legging lacings, and the like...."

"We didn't talk about such things. They were too horrible and obscene even for hardened veterans...It is too preposterous to think that men could actually live and fight for days and nights on end under such terrible conditions and not be driven insane...To me the war was insanity." (294)

The Wilhelm Gustloff

As WWII ground along toward its bloody end, other massive acts of brutality became commonplace, often unnoticed and unremarked by anyone other than their victims.

As German civilian refugees flooded westward, fleeing the Russian offensive into East Prussia in the bitter winter of 1945, many gathered at the port of Gdynia, praying that they might somehow gain sea passage to the west. On 30 January, the German cruise ship *Wilhelm Gustloff* finally departed Gdynia, unescorted, with over 8,000 refugees and noncombatants packed into her bowels. Within hours, a Russian submarine fired a salvo of three torpedoes into her side, at point blank range. Disaster followed as the ship began to sink in the icy sea:

> The German torpedo boat T-36 was the only vessel to render immediate assistance. It closed the scene in time to pick up 252 survivors. Many even among those who had found places in lifeboats froze to death before other rescuers arrived at daybreak. A naval petty officer who boarded one boat full of corpses the next morning found an unidentified baby, blue with cold but still breathing. He adopted it. The child became one of just 949 know survivors of the greatest maritime disaster in history, its 7,000 dead far outstripping those of the *Titanic, Lusitania, Laconia.* Yet, amid global tragedy on the scale of 1945, the horrors of the *Wilhelm Gustloff* remain known only to some Germans and a few historians. (Hastings, Retribution 287)

Brutality: The Bizarre Small Scale

Other acts of brutality were relatively small in scale, but nonetheless bizarre, when viewed through the lens of a civilized world.

A Snowy Christmas Scene

Stephan Ambrose describes several incidents that took place around Christmas, 1944, during the Battle of the Bulge: "On Christmas Day, Pvt. Louis Potts of the 26th Division was fired on while attending a wounded soldier. He stayed in the snow-covered field and went to work on another casualty. This time the German sniper got him in the forehead." (Ambrose, Citizen 315)

In the course of that same battle an American paratrooper, Frank Brumbaugh, came across a snow-covered field where the bodies of seventy fellow American soldiers, POWs of the Germans when they died, lay frozen in their death throes. They had been mowed down in cold blood days before:

> An hour or so later, he saw some paratroopers who had a bunch of Germans wearing either U.S. jump boots or infantry combat boots, obviously stolen from captive,

[37]

wounded, or dead Americans. The American paratroopers shot those wearing combat boots out of hand, on the grounds that if they had taken them from wounded or captured GIs, they may have caused injury or death, because the snow was deep, the weather bitter cold.

Those German captives found wearing U.S. parachute boots were made to remove the boots and socks, role their trousers above their knees, and march around in the snow until their feet were totally frozen and they could no longer feel a knife prick, nor walk." The prisoners were sent back to field hospitals, where both feet had to be amputated. (Ambrose, Citizen 356)

Viet Nam Redo: 3

Intense, continuous combat can very quickly harden and brutalize those involved. An excerpt from Ronald Glasser's *365 Days,* describing the end of a bloody 'Search and Destroy' mission in Viet Nam:

A cobra swept in, running down the whole length of the nearby hedgerow, cutting it apart with mini guns. The company charging through the heat took the wood line. Stumbling through the bushes, they overran it, killing everyone they found. Panting, barely able to catch his breath, the platoon's RTO found a wounded NVA, his shoulder and thighs mashed by the mini guns. Unable to move, he lay there, his AK broken beside him. The RTO shot him through the face. (Glasser 99)

Even after the immediacy of the active fighting has died out, survivors most often find themselves both numb and oftentimes quietly, brutally enraged. The devastation through which they have just passed leaves little room, emotionally speaking, for joyous claims of victory:

That afternoon the Americans, slinging their weapons, began counting bodies. The brass flew in, and to show how pleased they were, OK'd a policy of claiming a kill for every weapon found, even without a body. The exhausted troops, eighteen and nineteen-year old kids, ignored the congratulations and simply went on stacking the bodies, throwing them into countable piles. It was the chopper pilots, though, flying in and out of it, right through the center of an NVA regiment and losing nine choppers, who summed up the bitterness of what had happened. At dark of that last day of fighting, they flew in a CH-47 flying crane and slung a great cargo net below it. After the counting, they helped the troopers throw the NVA bodies into the net.

They filled the net quickly, and when it was filled, the crane, blowing up great clouds of dust, rose off the flat, pock-market paddy. When the net had cleared the ground, the crane spun slowly around its center and, carrying its dripping cargo, moved off to drop the bodies on the path of the retreating NVA. (Glasser 101)

A Murder at Baghdad University

Paul Rieckhoff, in his book *Chasing Ghosts,* describes, in clear, unflinching detail, random acts of brutality that occurred during the American occupation of Iraq. He describes one particularly harrowing incident, the killing of Specialist Jeffrey Wershow on the campus of Baghdad University, and the reverberating impact felt by he and his men in the days that followed.

Wershow was part of a security detail for a small group of American dignitaries who were visiting a crowded Baghdad University campus. During a break, Wershow was standing in line, waiting to buy a Coke. An Iraqi male walked up behind Wershow, shot him in the base of his skull, and then slipped away into the crowd. It was brutal, nothing more than a simple execution. Rieckoff describes the immediate aftermath:

The Commander in charge of security in the area, Lt. Col. Peter Jones, described the incident in the press as "an aberration."

Aberration, my ass. It was the same tactic used the day before in the killing of a British cameraman outside the Baghdad Museum. The close-quarters sneak attacks in crowded areas were terribly menacing. Maybe not for Lieutenant Colonels who never walked patrols, but for my enlisted grunts, who walked the streets every day, trying to win Iraqi hearts and minds, it was scary as hell. Any man shaking your right hand could shoot you in the face with the gun in his left....Tempers were high. Any time Iraqis tried to get close to us we'd shove them away. Each attack drove a larger wedge between us and them. (158-159)

Brutality: As Culture

Children of the Sun God

The racists controlling the Japanese government before the onset of WWII promoted the concept that, as the "Yamato" people, the Japanese were direct descendents of the Sun God, and were racially superior to all other peoples. Thus, they were not to be restrained by conventional rules when it came to conducting war. With the onset of WWII, the Japanese army, as it spread its flood of conquest across Asia, seemed to embrace a culture of brutality that had no limits. In his book, *War Without Mercy,* John Dower describes this phenomenon:

> Their atrocities frequently were so grotesque, and flaunted in such a macabre manner, that it is not surprising they were interpreted as being an expression of deliberate policy and a calculated exhibition of some perverse 'national character.' What else was one supposed to make, for example, of the 'friendly contest' between two officers in late 1937, avidly followed in some Japanese newspapers, to see who would be the first to cut down 150 Chinese with his samurai sword; or of the rape and murder of nuns in the streets of Hong Kong; or of the corpses of tortured Englishmen hanging from trees in Malaya, with their severed genitals in their mouths; or

of the water torture of old missionaries in Korea and Japan, who were then repatriated to tell their tales? (42)

Japanese/German Racial Superiority

The noted historian, Niall Ferguson, draws striking similarities between the attitudes toward racial eradication held by the two Axis allies, the Germans in Russia and the Japanese in China:

> It is no coincidence that both the Germans and the Japanese spoke of those they conquered as less than human; the term used for bedbugs in Manchuria-"Nanking vermin" --- tells its own story. "The Chinese people," wrote General Sakai Ryu, the Chief of Staff of the Japanese forces in North China in 1937, "are bacteria infesting world civilization." (Ferguson 473)

On a smaller scale, the fanaticism engendered in German youth by the ideal of racial and moral superiority, constantly preached over the years by the Nazi party, began to bear increasingly bitter fruit as the war descended into its final weeks. The most ardent of these indoctrinated youth enlisted in the SS, Hitler's favored legion. Their fanaticism would manifest a bitter harvest to the very end:

> On April 27, the 12th US Armored Division approached Landsberg-am-Lech, west of Munich. There was a Wehrmacht unit and a Waffen SS unit in the town. The Wehrmacht commander decided to withdraw across the Lech River. The SS commander wanted to fight. The regular officer told him to do as he wished, but the Wehrmacht troops were getting out of there. When the civilians saw the Wehrmacht soldiers leaving, they hung out white sheets. The sight infuriated the SS. "In their rage," Lt. Julius Bernstein related, "they went from house to house and dragged outside whomever they found and hanged them from the nearest tree or lamp post. As we rode into Landsberg, we found German

civilians hanging from trees like ripe fruit." (Ambrose, Citizen 463-464)

Russian Revenge

The Russian army, as it thrust further into East Prussia in the winter of 1945, was officially encouraged to take revenge upon everything German:

"Comrades! You have now reached the borders of East Prussia, and you will now tread that ground which gave birth to the fascist monsters who devastated our cities and homes, slaughtered our sons and daughters, our brothers and sisters, our wives and mothers. The most inveterate of those brigands and Nazis sprang from East Prussia. For many years they have held power in Germany, inspiring its foreign invasions and directing its genocides of alien peoples."

In the days before the Red Army crossed the border, political officers held meetings explicitly designed to promote hatred of the enemy, discussing such themes as "How shall I avenge myself on our German occupiers?" and "An eye for an eye." Later, when orders came from Moscow to adopt a less savage attitude towards Germans, to encourage surrenders, it was far too late to change an ethos cultivated over years of struggle. "Hatred for the enemy had become the most important motivation for our men," writes a Russian historian. "Almost every Soviet soldier possessed some personal reason to seek vengeance." (Hastings, Retribution 267-268)

Brutality: POWs

The treatment received by POWs is dramatically influenced by the nature and intensity of the combat that takes place immediately before capture. Critical to the fate of the POW is one supremely important question: has the capturing unit suffered the loss of a beloved comrade(s) in the action that just ended?

This is a subject area that is almost always omitted from 'official' histories. To shine a revealing light into this dark corner would surely tarnish the honor and beauty of "the noble cause", whichever one that it might be.

Well, not me… but other guys did…

Stephen Ambrose, whose distinguished career as a military scholar and historian spans decades, has the following interesting observations:

> Both the American and the German army outlawed the shooting of unarmed prisoners. Both sides did it, frequently, but no court-martials were ever convened for men charged with shooting prisoners. It is a subject everyone agreed should not be discussed, and no records were kept. Thus all commentary on the subject is anecdotal.
>
> I've interviewed well over 1,000 combat veterans. Only one of them said he shot a prisoner, and he added that while he felt some remorse he would do it again. Perhaps as many as one-third of the veterans I've talked to, however, related incidents in which they saw other GIs shooting unarmed German prisoners who had their hands up. The general attitude was expressed by Lt. Tom Gibson of the 101st Airborne, who told me in graphic detail of the murder of ten German POWs by an American airborne officer – he shot them while they were digging a ditch and were under guard. Gibson commented: "I firmly believe that only a combat soldier has the right to judge another combat soldier. Only he knows how hard it is to retain his sanity, to do his duty and to survive with some semblance of honor. You have to learn to forgive others, and yourself, for some of the things that are done."(Ambrose, Citizen 352)

In the dessert: "No Prisoners!"

T. E. Lawrence, the famed 'Lawrence of Arabia' won acclaim fighting the Turks with his Arab allies in WWI. He speaks to the issue of POWs with remarkable honestly and directness in his autobiography, *The Seven Pillars of Wisdom.*

Combat Veterans

Toward the end of the war, Lawrence and his small Arab army were driving a retreating Turkish column back towards Damascus, when they came upon the smoldering ruins of the Arab village of Tafas. The Turks, in a fit of unbound brutality, had totally destroyed the village, burning, raping and butchering all the villagers that they could get their hands on, including children, a pregnant woman and the elderly. As it happened, riding next to Lawrence was Tallal, both a fearless Arab warrior and a trusted lieutenant. Tallal was also a native of Tafas:

> Tallal has seen what we had seen. He gave one moan like a hurt animal; then rode to the upper ground and sat there a while on his mare, shivering and looking fixedly after the Turks....then he suddenly seemed to take hold of himself, for he dashed his stirrups into the mare's flanks and galloped headlong, bending low and swaying in the saddle, right at the main body of the enemy. (Lawrence 632)

Frozen in place, Lawrence and his army watched in silence as Tallal plunged down a long slope, closing to within several lengths of the Turkish rearguard before he and his mare were cut down in a hail of rifle and machinegun fire. Lawrence broke the silence as he screamed his command; "No prisoners! No prisoners!"

In a blaze of passion, Lawrence and his army engulfed the Turkish column, splitting it into three isolated sections before setting about their grim work of slaughter:

> In a madness born of the horror of Tafas, we killed and killed, even blowing in the heads of the fallen and the animals; as though their death and running blood could slake our agony...just one group of Arabs, who had not heard our news, took prisoner of the last two hundred men of the central section. Their respite was short. I had gone up to learn why it was....they said nothing in the moments before we opened fire. At last their heap ceased moving...we mounted again and rode slowly home. (633)

[44]

Kill, then Surrender

It is a pattern that is easily recognizable, regardless of the particular war: POWs are treated brutally in the heat of battle and/or after the death of a beloved fellow soldier. The following incident took place during the final days of WWII in Europe. As American infantry units pushed further eastward into Germany, a few die-hard German soldiers refused to recognize that the war was lost:

Pemberton's unit kept advancing. "The Krauts always shot up all their ammo and then surrendered," he remembered. Hoping to avoid such nonsense, in one village the CO sent a Jewish private who spoke German forward with a white flag, calling out to the German boys to surrender. "They shot him up so bad that after it was over the medics had to slide a blanket under his body to take him away. Then the Germans started waving their own white flag. Single file, eight of them emerged from a building, hands up. They were very cocky. They were about 20 feet from me when I saw the leader suddenly realize he still had a pistol in his shoulder holster. He reached into his jacket with two fingers to pull it out and throw it away."

One of our guys yelled, "Watch it! He's got a gun!" and came running up shooting and there were eight Krauts on the ground shot up but not dead. They wanted water but not one gave them any. I never felt bad about it although I'm sure civilians would be horrified. But these guys asked for it. If we had not been so tired and frustrated and keyed up and mad about our boys they shot up, it never would have happened. But a lot of things happen in war and both sides know the penalties." (Ambrose, Citizen 440)

Gerald Linderman, a Professor of History at the University of Michigan, addresses the stress of battle in great detail in his seminal book, *The World Within War.*

In the following passage, he quotes GIs who witnessed firsthand the fate of POWs, especially those who surrendered shortly after intense combat:

> Even in hopeless situations…the Germans would usually fight to the last, refusing to surrender. (Then) when their ammunition was gone, they were ready to give up and ask for mercy (but because) many American lives had been lost in this delay, our troops often killed Germans…
>
> Individual Germans to whom GIs thought they could trace specific American deaths often provoked similarly lethal reactions. Just after his unit crossed the Rhine, Frank Irgang watched American soldiers beat to death with his own weapon a persistent German machine gunner who "…was known to have inflicted several casualties upon us." (Linderman 111-112)

Two incidents, occurring over two decades and two continents apart, have a self-similar ring of tragedy about them. The first incident took place in the winter of 1944.

A Tardy Surrender: WWII

Pvt. Edward Webber of the 47th Infantry Regiment described a gruesome, but hardly unique, incident. He was advancing on a damaged German tank. The crew had ceased firing its machine gun, opened the turret, and was waving a white flag. Webber and his buddies moved forward. The machine gun began firing again – probably by some young fanatic who refused to give up. The rest of Webber's squad fired back. "The crew came pouring out of the bottom escape hatch," Webber said. "They were hollering '*Nicht schiessen! Nicht schiessen!*' But by this time we were in an infuriated rage. The crewmen were lined up on their knees and an angry soldier walked along behind them and shot each in the back of the head. The last to die was a young, blond-headed teenager who was rocking back and forth on his knees, crying and urinating down both trouser legs. He had pictures of his family spread on the ground before him. Nevertheless, he was shot in the back of the head and pitched forward like a sack of potatoes." (Ambrose, Citizen 352)

A Nasty Surrender: Viet Nam

Robert Mason, a helicopter pilot in Viet Nam assigned a mission to pick up NVA prisoners, describes the scene he encountered after flying into a remote combat LZ:

Twenty-one men lay trussed in a row, ropes at their ankles, hands bound under their backs --- North Vietnamese prisoners. A sergeant stood at the first prisoner's feet, his face twisted with anger. The North Vietnamese prisoner stared back, unblinking. The sergeant pointed a .45 at the man. He kicked the prisoner's feet suddenly. The shock of the impact jostled the prisoner inches across the earth. The sergeant fired the .45 into the prisoner's face. The prisoner's head bounced off the ground like a ball slapped from above, then flopped back into the gore that had been his brains. The sergeant turned to the next prisoner in the line. "He tried to get away," said a voice at my side."

"He can't get away; he's tied!"

"He moved. He was trying to get away."

The next prisoner said a few hurried words in Vietnamese as the sergeant stood over him. When the sergeant kicked his feet, the prisoner closed his eyes. A bullet shook his head.

"It's murder!" I hissed to the man at my side.

"They cut off Sergeant Rocci's cock and stuck it in his mouth. And five of his men," said the voice. "After they spent the night slowly shoving knives into their guts. If you had been there to hear the screams…They screamed all night. This morning they were all dead, all gagged with their cocks. This isn't murder; it's justice."

Another head bounced off the ground. The shock wave hit my body.

"They sent us to pick up twenty-one *prisoners*," I pleaded.

"You'll get'em. They'll just be dead, is all." (Mason 309)

The Mid-town Massacre: Iraq

On April 3, 2003, elements of the US 3rd Armored Division found themselves locked in a desperate, five-hour firefight just east of the Baghdad airport in an area called 'Ambush Alley'. At first it was touch and go for the troops, until they could bring their superior firepower to bear. The fighting spread wider and wider as it cranked up in both violence and intensity. Rumor had it that more than fifty Syrian fighters had clustered there and were determined to either kill the invading 'infidels' or to die trying. Before it was over there were confirmed reports of "bodies piled in the streets."

The prospect of taking POWs was particularly troublesome that day:

As they (US troops) assessed what remained of the office building, a suicide attacker wearing an explosive vest ran toward a squad further up the street. He detonated himself before he reached the squad but shrapnel struck a captain in his arm and his hand. "That's when the gloves came off," one soldier reported later. All combatants taken prisoner were thenceforth treated as potential suicide bombers….the battle's field colonel aimed his pistol at a combatant lying on the ground who he suspected (falsely) of concealing a live grenade and shot him. (Boal, *Playboy* May, 2004)

Specialist Richard Davis was one of the American soldiers fighting for his life that day in Ambush Alley. Three months later he would return stateside with his unit to Ft. Benning, Georgia. Within forty-eight hours of his return he would be dead, murdered by fellow soldiers from his company. The story of his death is portrayed in the film, *The Valley of Elah*. Also portrayed in the film is his brutal

[48]

behavior toward a wounded Iraqi POW on the day of the Mid-town Massacre. This was seemingly bizarre behavior for a young man who, by all accounts, was a decent, standup guy before Iraq:

> Later, back at Ft. Benning, attempting to put Davis' behavior in context, a fellow soldier said, "You know, *it's not like they tell you,* the Geneva Convention, and all that. When you're in a fight, you don't try to take prisoners or help the wounded. You finish people and keep moving. Tap-tap, two in the chest. At least, that's how we did it." (Boal, *Playboy* 2004)

This is the dark, painful stuff that we Combat Vets carry home with us. None of it fits well with images of handsome uniforms, sparkling medals and "heroes all."

But it's a brutal truth that the larger society must face to even begin to understand the experience of the Combat Veteran.

On this note we will end *Part I: What They Didn't Tell You.*

Combat Veterans

PART II: The Spiral

The Spiral: An Introduction

In *Part I* we focused on important pieces of the picture they didn't tell you about before you got into combat.

Now, we're going to take a closer look at what happens to each of us as individuals as we struggle in the face of life-threatening experiences.

For those of you who have survived combat, some details of what follows will be very familiar. You will also be introduced to other aspects that will most likely be both new and insightful.

By reading what follows, your loved ones will gain a new level of understanding about your journey. This process has helped many Combat Vets and their families bridge the yawning gap in experience that so often seems to be both insurmountable and isolating.

To guide our exploration, we will introduce *The Spiral*, a model that maps the changes experienced by the individual as they struggle through their immersion in combat. We will look at the three stages of the Spiral and how they together describe the psychological, emotional and spiritual costs that accumulate over time.

We will include the personal experiences of Combat Vets from many different wars (WWI, WWII, Korea, Viet Nam, Iraq and Afghanistan) as a means of illustrating specific examples of each stage of the Spiral. Although the details of these various settings vary greatly, it is clear that the passage through the Spiral is the same in each.

The foundation of *The Spiral* is built upon decades of reading and research. The model itself weaves together a collection of profound insights drawn from the work of some very wise people.

It is also the outgrowth of my quest to understand and come to grips with my own experience in combat.

This is a dark journey, but one well worth taking. It is a journey that moves us toward the light of knowledge and personal healing.

An Honorable Truth-Sayer: Malarkey

Sgt. Donald Malarkey was one of the most respected members of the "Band of Brothers." His company, the famed E Company of the 506th PIC of the 101st Airborne, jumped into Normandy on D-Day, June 6th, 1944. The opening sequence of his autobiography, *Easy Company Soldier*, follows:

> Bastogne, Belgium
> January 3, 1945
> One shot.
> That's all it would take, I figure, as I warmed my hands around the campfire with a few other shivering soldiers. One shot and the frozen hell of Belgium's Ardennes Forest would be over for me.
> It was January, 1945, seven months since me and the guys…had jumped into the dark sky over Normandy. Now, a handful of us E Company guys were numb from the war, death, and bitter cold and snow. In the flames flickering light, I looked down at my boots, wrapped in burlap bags and purposely dipped in water so they'd freeze and keep my feet warmer.
> One shot and those damn feet would never be cold again. One shot and the sight of Joe Toye and Bill Guarnere lying in the snow, each missing a leg, would never haunt me again.
> Why Toye? Why not the SOB who I'd seen a few days ago slicing the fingers off the dead Germans so to get their rings…
> And why Guarnere? He gets it trying to save Joe. The Germans are raining down artillery shells like a Fourth of July

show gone wrong, and Bill sees Joe out there trying to get up and so runs across the snow to save his buddy. Sort of like one swimmer trying to help another swimmer who's drowning. And, boom, both end up drowning…

One shot.

I looked at the flames and fingered the pistol, a P38 I'd picked up from a German we'd taken prisoner in Holland. One shot and I'd be back (home). Not a shot to the head, though a few soldiers were known to do that, too. But one in the foot. (Malarkey 1-3)

It is striking that Don Malarkey, a man of unquestioned courage, would choose to open his autobiography with such a revealing, piercing look into his own heart. His is the heart of a Combat Vet who has had enough, who has passed downward through the Spiral into the final stage of Exhaustion.

He does great honor to himself (and to all of us who have been there) by speaking with such unflinching honesty.

The Foundation of *the Spiral*

So we need to ask the following questions:

-How does this journey down the Spiral that ends in Exhaustion take place?

-What does each stage of the Spiral look like?

-How does it drive a motivated, volunteer soldier (like Malarkey) to a place where he's ready to do almost anything to get out of combat?

-What are the keys that trigger the Spiral, and how do they affect individuals differently?

-Where does it end?

-And how do we get back to sanity, to safe harbor from there?

-How do we "Bring Home" the process of the Spiral?

To seek answers to these questions, we'll first review some historical trends. Then we'll follow up by exploring new research that offers insight into the critical keys in the Spiral process.

First, let's check some facts.

Combat Veterans

Over the last four centuries, the old myth of unlimited physical, mental and emotional courage began to slowly die. It suddenly evaporated in the cauldron of the modern battlefield, beginning with WWI.

The new intensity, frequency, and depth of modern combat quickly sent casualty figures rocketing skyward. Soon after WWI began, the military establishment in the Western democracies began to research battlefield stress and its effect upon the individual soldier. In the opening months of the war British soldiers exhibiting psychiatric symptoms had been considered 'shirkers', and were sometimes shot for cowardice. By the end of 1916, however, the reality had changed. The British high command had found it necessary to set up special psychiatric centers for each of their individual army groups. The mass of war torn soldiers being generated by the horror of trench warfare was simply too large to send to the firing squads.

Twenty-five years later, an important study conducted by the US Army (early in WWII) concluded that "there was no such a thing as getting used to combat" (Holmes 215). The Army researchers found that it is the intensity and duration of combat that wear the individual combatant down, just like piling hard miles onto a set of tires eventually ends in failure. Not only do soldiers become combat ineffective, they also became cautious and jittery to the point that they were a liability to their unit and demoralized less experienced soldiers.

Combat exhaustion also occurred in the armies of Germany and Russia during WWII. In both cases, it was dealt with black and white brutality: to falter in the face of combat meant either immediate execution or assignment to a penal assault battalion (which was essentially a death penalty in a different form). Combat exhaustion took an even greater toll in these armies because soldiers were never treated, never given a brief respite to heal and then the chance to return to their unit.

From our earlier discussion of the evolution of War, let's review the following important facts:

- Over time, modern weapons have continued to become much more powerful, varied, far-ranging, and destructive.

- Both the frequency and the intensity of actual combat in a modern war are both much greater than in past wars.
- The size and shape of the battlefield have vastly expanded with each new generation of weaponry. The breadth and depth of the killing zone (the area in which a soldier is at risk of dying) continued to expand as it kept pace with the increased complexity of the battlefield.

The killing zone was never a good place to be, even at Agincourt, when it was relatively small: only two hundred yards wide. But because it was so small, it was also a relatively easy place from which to escape, even for combatants.

By the time of the battle of Waterloo in 1814, the killing zone had grown to over a half a mile wide. By 1916, during the battle of the Somme in WWI, it was upwards of five miles wide and several miles deep, thus able to collect tens of thousands of combatants in its deadly grasp (a huge transformational growth from Agincourt).

As the killing zone continued to grow ever larger, it became more difficult for combatants to get a respite, a chance to drop their guard and shut off the stress, even momentarily. The killing zone in Viet Nam eventually encompassed the entire country, even engulfing the American embassy in Saigon. And with the emergence of the IED, incredibly powerful truck bombs, rockets and mortars, every square foot of Iraq became potentially lethal (including the Green Zone in Baghdad).

In stark contrast, Wellington and most of his commanders spent the evening before the battle of Waterloo waltzing with satin-gowned ladies in a resplendent, crystal palace in Brussels. So, in a little over a century, the face of War had changed dramatically:

> The crucial point here is that, while wars were often long, battles were short and relatively infrequent. If modern estimates of a man's tolerance of days of combat are applied to the soldiers of the Napoleonic period, then most of them would have fought for years without amassing as many combat days as, say, a British or American soldier in Italy in 1944-45.

Nevertheless, sudden and traumatic shocks – like the concentrated gunfire at Zorndorf or Waterloo – might drain the well of courage dry at a single draught. Sieges, too, whose conditions often approximated to the dangerous stalemate on the Western Front in 1914-18, seemed to bruise men's tolerance more than battles in open field. (Holmes 216)

Ernst Junger, a German infantry officer with extensive combat experience during WWI, offers this insight into modern combat: "It is a mistake to believe that soldiers toughen and become more brave in the course of a war. What they gain in technique, in knowing how to deal with the enemy, they lose in nervous exhaustion." (Holmes 218-219)

Today, military institutions have finally accepted the fact that there are real, predictable limits that impose themselves onto the durability of a soldier exposed to combat.

Let's now take a look at how the individual soldier reacts to the powerful emotion currents that are always flowing in the killing zone. These are powerful currents that are flowing either just below the surface or exploding with an unavoidable fury. After that we'll take a look at how groups of humans respond to extreme stress in both the civilian setting and as combatants in war.

The Amygdala

(This next section reviews in specific detail some complex aspects of the brain and the process whereby the brain reacts to perceived threat. If these details don't interest you, fast-forward to the 'Take-away' summary on page 59).

In his groundbreaking book, *The Emotional Brain*, Joseph LeDoux describes the intricate and complex inner workings of the human brain. Researchers had just recently discovered some startling new aspects to the role of the amygdala (a relatively small, almond shaped section of the brain) plays in the processing of emotionally potent stimuli:

Information about external stimuli reaches the amygdala by way of direct pathways from the thalamus (the low road) as well as by way of pathways from the thalamus to the cortex to the amygdala. The direct thalamo-amygdala path is shorter and thus a faster transmission route than the pathway from the thalamus through the cortex to the amygdala. However, because the direct pathway bypasses the cortex, it is unable to benefit from cortical processing. As a result, it can only provide the amygdala with a crude representation of the stimulus. It is thus a quick and dirty processing pathway. The direct pathway allows us to begin to respond to potentially dangerous stimuli before we fully know what the stimulus is. This can be very useful in dangerous situations. (LeDoux 164)

Translated into layman's terms, our brains are wired so that a primary 'hotline' runs directly from our sensory organs (eyes, ears, skin, smell, taste) to the amygdala. That hotline bypasses our cortex, the area of the brain where we 'think' or 'reason'. A second, slower 'hotline' runs from our senses to the cortex, and only then to the amygdala. So, by the time we've given 'thought' to a given stimuli, the amygdala has already been stimulated and has reacted. LeDoux places the amygdala right in the center of the whole process. He calls it "a Hub in the Wheel of Fear":

The amygdala is like the hub of a wheel. It receives low-level inputs from sensory-specific regions of the thalamus, higher level information from sensory s-specific cortex, and still higher level (sensory independent) information about the general situation from the hippocampal formation. Through such connections, the amygdala is able to process the emotional significance of individual stimuli as well as complex situations. The amygdala is, in essence, involved in the appraisal of emotional meaning. It is where the trigger stimuli do their triggering. (LeDoux 168)

Being the "Hub in the Wheel," the activation of the amygdala reverberates throughout the entire body:

> ...activation of the amygdala results in the automatic activation of networks that control the expression of a variety of responses: species-specific behaviors (freezing, fleeing, fighting, facial expressions), autonomic nervous system (ANS) responses (changes in blood pressure and heart rate, piloerection, sweating), and hormonal responses (release of stress hormones, like adrenaline and adrenal steroids, as well as a host of peptides, into the bloodstream). The ANS and hormonal responses can be considered together as visceral responses --- responses of the internal organs and glands (the viscera). When these behavioral and visceral responses are expressed, they create signals in the body that return to the brain. (LeDoux 291)

It is interesting that LeDoux describes (in very clinical terms) a whole range of the very same reactions that Vets report when exposed to combat. The difference, of course, is that he describes "responses of internal organs and glands" while Vets would describe a pounding heart, emptying of the bowels, a cold sweat, shortness of breath and peeing in their pants.

Finally, LeDoux summarizes the overarching impact of emotions on the brain:

> When we are in the throes of emotion, it is because something important, perhaps life-threatening, is occurring, and much of the brain's resources are brought to bear on the problem. Emotions create a flurry of activity all devoted to one goal. Thoughts, unless they trigger emotional systems, don't do this. We can daydream while doing other things, like reading or eating, and go back and forth between the daydream and the other activities. But when faced with danger or other challenging emotional situations, we don't have time to kill nor do we have spare mental resources. The whole self gets

absorbed in the emotion. As Klaus Scherer has argued, emotions cause a mobilization and synchronization of the brain's activities. (LeDoux 299-300)

Take-away:

Here are several important concepts gleaned from LeDoux's work which will be very useful as we move forward into our exploration of the Spiral:

A.   The pre-conscious "Low Road" reaction to perceived danger is much, much faster than the "High Road" thoughtful reaction.

B.   This "Low Road" reaction activates and synchronizes the brain's activities. This is a mixed bag, however: when the whole system goes to instant alert, there is a price is to be paid. Part of the cost is that our clarity of perception becomes poorer (we hear less clearly, we see less accurately, often getting tunnel vision, we feel less grounded and secure). Our ability to think clearly and rationally tends to decrease dramatically.

These are the reactions that most Vets experience when they are first exposed to combat. We will discuss them in detail later.

Survivorship: When your plane goes down

In her tantalizing new book, *The Unthinkable: Who Survives When Disaster Strikes-and Why*, Amanda Ripley builds upon the work of LeDoux in some very interesting ways. She has also done a remarkable job of drawing together research that offers insight into our subject:

> Today most people who study decision making agree that human beings are not rational...people rely on two different systems: the intuitive and the analytical. The intuitive

[59]

system is automatic, fast, emotional and swayed heavily by experiences and images. The analytical is the ego to the brain's id: logical, contemplative and pragmatic. (Ripley 32)

So, when we are faced with what appears to be catastrophic risk, our first reaction is intuitive and highly emotional. Depending upon the circumstances, such a response sometimes serves us well, helping to insure our survival. At other times, this same reaction sets us up for tragic mistakes.

Ripley has created a three-step model to describe the pathway that the individual (as well as the larger group) passes through when faced with such a crisis:

1. **Denial**
2. **Deliberation**
3. **Decision**

First, we will consider each of these steps as it applies to a crisis in civilian life. Later, we'll look at how these steps apply to Combat Vets as they are exposed to battle.

Denial:

For the vast majority of humans, the initial reaction to a potentially catastrophic crisis is Denial. It is the response that most all of us have stumbled through at least once in our lives: "No! This can't be happening!" Individuals as well as whole groups can get stuck in Denial, literally refusing to believe their own senses as a violent or physically dangerous event unfolds before them. The resulting 'deer in the headlights' response is potentially deadly. The problem is compounded because Denial blocks our ability to grasp the simple reality of the situation, much less begin to fix it.

In our previous discussion of the amygdala and LeDoux's "emotional brain," we learned about the flooding activated by the amygdala. It does a great job of alerting us to imminent danger. **But it also severely decreases our ability to perceive clearly as well as our ability to think clearly.**

For example, many reports surfaced after the two separate, sequential airplane attacks on the World Trade Center on 9/11 that many occupants of both Towers responded to the first, initial attack on Tower 1 by doing… nothing! The situation was exacerbated in Tower 2 by a public address announcement by a Port Authority official prompting everyone to stay in place. Nonetheless, in 20/20 hindsight, it is pretty amazing that folks gazed out the windows of Tower 2, watching Tower 1 burning, and remained totally passive!

But even in Tower 1, where the impact of the airplane had clearly been felt throughout the building, people stayed put:

> On average, Trade Center survivors waited six minutes before heading downstairs…from a study of nearly nine hundred survivors. (The average would likely be higher if those who died had been able to respond to the survey). Some waited as long as forty-five minutes…many called relatives and friends. About one thousand individuals took the time to shut down their computers. (Ripley 8-9)

Deliberation:

As the dense, foggy confusion of initial Denial begins to clear, the process of Deliberation begins: "My world has just turned to shit, so what now?" The difficulty that we suddenly face is that we're trying to problem-solve while working with a diminished capacity to sense and to think. The amygdala has done its job, sounding the alarm, shocking our system into a high state of alert but at a great cost. Numerous studies have documented that almost all people under extreme stress experience a profoundly altered visual capacity, most often in the form of tunnel vision. On top of that, most folks experiencing this kind of stress-shock seem to be unable to hear clearly, because external sound either seems to be muted or seems to be extraordinarily loud: "Stress hormones are like hallucinogenic drugs. Almost no one gets through an ordeal…without experiencing some kind of altered reality."(Ripley 64)

As another classic example, Ripley cites the phenomena wherein passengers on a just-crashed airplane tend to stay frozen in their seats after impact. Even after the plane has come to a complete stop and even though the danger of fire is eminent, the vast majority remain frozen in their seats. Groups of people stuck in this stage tend to act as an immobile herd, clinging passively to one another, despite staring directly into the face of impending death or disaster.

As it turns out, after-the-fact reports document that just the tiniest bit of preparation pays huge dividends. Study after study has found that preparation of even the most minimal amounts favored survival (such as taking the time to determine where the exit rows are on the airplane). More extensive preparation (as occurs in the training of police officers, firefighters, emergency medical personnel) create an opportunity for a reflexive, trained response that bypasses the confusion of Denial and Deliberation, triggering Decision instead.

Ripley (and many others) point to the work of Rick Rescorla, a Viet Nam Combat Veteran, who was working as the Director of Security for Morgan Stanley at the Twin Towers on 9/11. He achievements on that tragic day serve as a classic example of such a life saving bypass.

In the wake of the 1993 truck bombing in the parking garage of the World Trade Center, Rescorla realized that things had to change. He confronted the Morgan Stanley senior management with the reality that, as the Center's largest tenant, the company must be better prepared for the inevitable "next time" attack. As a result of his impassioned, professional approach, Rescorla was given free rein to mandate fire drills and regular evacuation training for Morgan Stanley's 2,700 employees. Thus, in the face of the 9/11 attack, the extensive training mandated by Rescorla served as an automatic override (bypassing Denial, Deliberation); the vast bulk of the Morgan Stanley staff were able to immediately move to and act from the Decision stage. As a consequence, on 9/11, Morgan Stanley lost only thirteen of 2700 employees. Among those lost, sadly enough, was Rick Rescorla himself, who chose to remain in the building, helping others try to escape until the building finally collapsed.

Decision:

We've just explored the classic situation whereby both the individual and a very large group can move quickly and safely from Deliberation to Decision. As is often the case, Decision in a group setting can be triggered by a single individual who acts decisively to propel others toward survival. Given the documented passivity of passengers in a downed airliner, flight attendants are now trained to yell instructions to passengers in a loud, intrusive voice: "Move to the exits now!!"

Countless other reports of critical incidents, from restaurant fires to shipwrecks, support the principle that a single leader can effectively move large groups by issuing clear, simple commands that break the deadly, frozen grasp of Deliberation.

Combat: Denial to Deliberation to Decision

Denial in Combat

A Combat Vet who had recently returned from Iraq described his first firefight to me this simply: "Then it hit me: they're really trying to kill me!"

For those of us who have survived the experience, the realization that someone is seriously trying to kill you is a life-changing event. A quick and clear reaction is most often critical to survival. Some soldiers freeze, stuck in Denial, not yet ready to grasp the reality of the situation. Again, the amygdala has, of course, kicked into high gear, sending shock waves throughout the body. When the reality finally hits home, many Vets describe the experience as shocking and disorienting, often accompanied by a set of overwhelming physical reactions.

On the battlefield, Denial is often a fatal response, if not bypassed immediately. The sudden realization, "This is for real!" floods your system with raw, largely unfocused energy. Clarity of perception (seeing and hearing especially) is dramatically diminished as is the ability to think clearly (remember the amygdala above). Reflexively, many individuals tend to simply freeze. An American

infantry officer describes a frozen moment in one of his first
encounters with the hailstorm of combat:

> "Time appeared to stand still….My mind seemed to
> reject the reality of what was happening, to say it was all make
> believe…One of our young lieutenants danced a rubber-legged
> jig as he twisted slowly, making the bullet hole between his
> eyes clearly visible. One moment our battalion chaplain and
> his assistant were kneeling beside their vehicle. The next
> moment they were headless, decapitated by an exploding shell
> as if by the stroke of a guillotine." (Ambrose, Citizen 191)

As a rule of thumb, it would be safe to assume that the vast
majority of Vets who manage to survive combat are able to get through
Denial very, very quickly. There are others, however, who don't
survive even their first baptism of fire because they are either
unwilling or unable to get up to speed fast enough.

During WWII, individual replacements sent into veteran
combat units had tough challenges ahead of them. They had to both
find their way on the battlefield and, at the same time, find some way
to fit in with the more experienced Combat Veterans:

> The replacements paid the cost. Often more than half
> became casualties within the first three days in the line. The
> odds were against a replacement's surviving long enough to
> gain recognition and experience. It was to the obvious benefit
> of the old boys to help the young kids, but nevertheless most
> veterans tried to avoid replacements. For one thing the new
> men tended to draw fire because they bunched up, talked too
> much and lit cigarettes at night. (Ambrose, Citizen 277)

In Viet Nam, soldiers and Marines new 'in-country' knew they
had a 365-day tour in front of them. As replacements, they were fed
piecemeal into combat units out in the field. They then had to find
some way to be integrated with experienced 'Short-timers'. The troops

who had a 'short' amount of time left in their tour before they were to be rotated home were proud to be 'Short-timers'.

As a result of this process, a whole new set of descriptive handles arose: the 'FNG' ('Fuckin' New Guy') or 'Fuckin' Cherry', the impersonal labels often used by the combat-wise Short-timers. Such impersonal labeling served as a way to distance themselves from replacements, who were yet to prove themselves dependable or trustworthy; to emphasize the inner connectedness of their shrinking circle of longtime survivors who were all 'real' people with names and value; and to underscore how close to the end of their trial by fire they had come. The negative spin also reflected the Short-timers resentment about how often the FNGs didn't listen to the voice of experience,

And, predictably, some of the FNGs never managed to get through Denial. They were either unwilling or unable to recognize and respond to the life-and-death gravity of the situation. Instead, some of them would immediately alienate more experienced Short-timers because their Denial would increase the risk level to all who were in close proximity.

My infantry platoon in Viet Nam received a perfectly flawed FNG: a new in-country replacement who prepared to go out on his first six-man night ambush by packing one of his two ammo pouches with a Kodak Instamatic camera (it fit his ammo pouch perfectly). Clearly, he thought carrying his camera was more important than the three clips of ammo (for his M-16 rifle) that he was leaving behind. He lasted less than a month because he never did get past the Denial.

By refusing to grasp the dangerous reality of the world of war, the FNG can linger in the relative comfort of Denial. A group of replacements who "bunched up, talked too much and lit cigarettes at night" gives us a perfect Denial profile. This passive herding instinct is deadly on a battlefield when they enemy is eagerly seeking targets of opportunity.

Leaving one-half of the basic load of ammunition behind in base camp in order to take a camera on a night ambush is just another layer of unreality. One of my Short-timers commented to me, as he wryly chuckled to himself, "And, shit, oh dear, Lieutenant, his little Kodak didn't even have a flash attachment!"

Deliberation in Combat

To summarize: survival on the battlefield can be broken down into a sequence of adaptations:

- First and foremost, the ability to pass very quickly through the deer-in-the-headlights shock of Denial
- Secondly, to move very, very rapidly through and beyond the uncertainty of Deliberation. This can be done by learning from more experienced combatants and by being a quick study who takes the immediate lessons of the battlefield to heart
- Finally, to achieve and maintain a decisive reflex that bypasses Denial and Deliberation on an ongoing basis

Without any question, this progression is dramatically accelerated by having the opportunity to follow the lead of more experienced Short-timers. Any replacement FNG who is able to quickly learn and integrate these hard-won survival skills immediately increases the odds of survival. Those without survival role models can acquire the necessary skills by focusing and staying attuned even when the learning curve starts to flatten out.

Even if the Denial stage passes quickly, Deliberation can hold a new combatant in its grasp longer than is good for one's health:

Soldiers who learned enough and lived long enough developed intuitive reactions to the dangers with which combat accosted them. Surviving combat soldiers developed what John Muirhead called a 'sensitivity learned from peril'. Reactions came faster and faster until they became automatic…'your body and mind react mechanically, performing their duties from trained habit as swiftly and efficiently as when you're more conscious of your acts….So, in assaults, an infantryman might always be looking, without consciousness of his constant calculation, for the next hole into which he could throw himself, and would, if suddenly brought under fire, find himself in it before he became aware that his mind had registered danger. (Linderman 60-61)

Some never get that far. Some remain stuck in Denial and Deliberation and relatively quickly become casualties in one form or another:

Capt. John Colby caught one of the essences of combat, the sense of total immediacy: "At this point, we had been in combat six days. It seemed like a year. In combat, one lives in the now and does not think much about yesterday or tomorrow"....Colby discovered that there was no telling who would break and when. His regimental CO was grossly incompetent, his battalion commander had run away from combat in his first day of action, and his company CO was a complete bust....(Colby's) company got caught in a combined mortar-artillery barrage. The men couldn't move forward, they couldn't fall back, and they couldn't stay where they were --- or so it appeared to the CO, who therefore had no orders to give, and was speechless. Colby went up to his CO to ask for orders. The CO shook his head and pointed to his throat. Colby asked him if he could make it back to the aid station on his own..." he leaped to his feet and took off. I never saw him again." (Ambrose, Citizen 61)

A dramatic scene in *Band of Brothers* depicts Capt. Winters, the Easy Company CO, initiating an attack (by himself, at first) on a company of German SS (over one hundred men) while they remain helplessly, fatally stuck in Deliberation. Winters describes the unfolding scene in his own words:

"The movements of the Germans seemed unreal to me. When they rose up, it seemed to be so slow, when they turned to look over their shoulders at me it was in slow motion, when they started to raise their rifles to fire at me, it was in slow, slow motion. I emptied the first clip (eight rounds) and, still

[67]

standing in the middle of the road, put in a second clip and, still shooting from the hip, emptied that clip into the mass." (Ambrose, Band 147-148)

Countless anecdotal instances, from many different wars, have described situations in which both individuals and groups avoid the need to act decisively by remaining frozen in Deliberation: Argentineans hiding in sleeping bags in the Falklands; Japanese soldiers hiding in the bottom of their foxhole; Viet Cong refusing to leave the illusionary safety their bunkers at Hoa Hoi are but a few examples. (Holmes 268)

Ripley labels this pattern of response as "the Disaster Default" (while underscoring the fact that not a lot of research has been done in this area) (Ripley 167-168).

To illustrate, she cites the example of Clay Violand, a student who survived the Virginia Tech killings in the spring of 2008. A deranged shooter (who eventually killed himself) burst into Violand's French classroom and began randomly shooting students. Violand survived by continuing to "play dead" while he heard the shooter pause and reload his handgun at least three times:"Of all the students in the French classroom that day, the only person not shot was Clay Violand... (he) was attacked by a lethal predator and he experienced a radical and involuntary survival response."(Ripley 170-171)

Given the process we've just discussed, Clay Violand's response would be described as anything but "involuntary" by the vast majority of Combat Veterans. To the contrary, if, on the battlefield, he were to respond to an extreme crisis with the same degree of total passivity, he would quickly find himself both isolated and doomed.

Decision in combat

Those Vets who manage to survive their initial exposures to combat are those who pass through Denial very quickly, seldom, if ever, get stuck in Deliberation and learn to move to the Decision mode in an instant. Again, countless instances from countless wars describe to us the process whereby experienced combatants reflexively, intuitively react to danger.

These reactions often seem to be preconscious. They become the manifestation of a sixth sense that grows stronger with experience and with repeated success at "dodging the bullet."

Like many other Combat Vets, I vividly remember the early warning signs that grew out of experience. In one instance, the hair on the back of my neck literally stood up as my small six-man patrol slowly approached a potentially lethal ambush site. We were all Short-timers, wired together in sync; not a word needed to be spoken as we carefully extricated ourselves, withdrawing to safety.

Instant, life-saving Decisions can manifest in the larger unit as well as the individual. The incident described above in which Capt. Winters leads elements of Easy Company in their assault on the German SS company (frozen in Deliberation) is an excellent example. Winters and his unit <u>as a whole</u>, confronting a potentially catastrophic situation, acted decisively, purposefully, collectively and rationally even in the face of what could have been emotionally terrifying odds.

Battlewise

The capacity to act decisively within a framework of hard-won survival skills is best described as being 'Battlewise.' This is the term used in the US Army's study of "combat efficiency" among soldiers fighting in Normandy in the summer of 1944. (Holmes 214)

This level of survivability is achieved by the average soldier after about ten days in combat. The shock they experienced in the initial exposure has passed; they no longer get stuck in indecision and react quickly to changing circumstance. The following thirty days or so is the period described in the study as "maximum efficiency." It is a relatively brief window of time in which the Battlewise combatant can be both a competent fighter and an asset to the unit. Much of the skill and efficiency that marks this period seems to manifest both reflexively and intuitively.

A Marine officer fighting in the South Pacific during WWII described battle-wisdom this way:

"When your senses are on alert you can feel dangers approach. On patrol through jungle trails where you are liable to meet Japs head-on, where they wait in ambush, where they bivouac, you can feel when they're near. A sharp, prickling sensation runs up your back; you slow down your patrol and approach with infinite caution and silence." (Linderman 62)

This level of competence comes with a high price tag. The repeated, unpredictable, violent triggering of our alarm system has many unintended consequences:"In other words, trauma creates such a searing impression on our brains that it feels, in retrospect, like it happened in slow motion." (Ripley 67).

This is exactly the phenomena described by Capt. Winters in his encounter with the German SS unit, stuck in Deliberation: "....when they started to raise their rifles to fire at me, it was in slow, slow motion...."

I experienced a similar sense of time distortion when reacting to a confrontation with a NVA soldier, armed with an AK-47, who suddenly emerged from a hedgerow within arm's length of me. As I was spinning around, I opened fire and killed him, I was struck by the surreal sensation that I was moving twice as fast as those around me, both friend and enemy alike. After emptying my M-16 into the NVA and the hedgerow, I grabbed another M-16 from the soldier immediately behind me (who hadn't moved, being frozen in Denial). As I sprayed the hedgerow with his rifle, I was shouting for my machinegun crew to come up, to add to my base of fire.

That sensation of elongated time no doubt helped save my life. That's the good news.

The bad news is that we pay a high price for this process: in fits and starts, we become more and more physically and psychologically worn down. As the amygdala gets triggered over and over again, as we repeatedly get instantly catapulted into that altered state of consciousness, our whole being is distorted. The wear and tear is accumulative, wearing us ragged around the edges. Each trigger requires a debit on our remaining, dwindling reserve of resiliency.

We'll discuss the specific details of this process below.

The Spiral of Combat

We now have all the concepts in place to make it possible for us to use the *Spiral* as a map. It can guide us as we explore in detail the process of change experienced by Combat Vets as they are immersed further and further into combat. To understand the many facets of the Spiral, we will again pay special attention to first-hand accounts of those who have struggled through and survived their passage into darkness.

We will once again draw extensively upon the work of Amanda Ripley, Gerald Linderman and Stephen Ambrose, whose collective insights form the foundations upon which this model is built.

To be able to grasp the complexity of the *Spiral*, we will explore it as a three-stage de-evolution, each stage following from and falling downward from the previous one.

Spiral I: Numbing/ Toughening

Numbing/Toughening

Combat Vets often look back in amazement at the infinite varieties of ugliness they encountered in their early exposure to the battlefield. For their emotional and psychological survival, they learn very quickly to numb themselves out. To be able to continue to function, they force themselves through and beyond the shock of death, beyond the stench of decaying bodies, to reach a place where their tender emotions are safely shut away. They are forced to learn to distance themselves from the suffering of friend and foe alike. Even the elation that some feel after surviving a near-miss with death eventually fades into a joyless, flat, matter of fact, I-didn't-die-this-time.

The process of *Toughening* proceeds hand in hand with the process of *Numbing*. By being emotionally insulated, Combat Vets can push themselves further than ever before, even in the face of numbing fear and horror. Because their soft emotions are inaccessible, they grow harder, more relentless, more black and white; sometimes merciless, vicious, punitive, vengeful, even fearless. For the vast majority, this is a bruising but necessary evolution.

(At the same time, there seems to be a very small minority, probably less than 10%, who really get energy out of this evolution. They're usually the ones who came into combat already numbed out; they don't need to toughen up by shutting away their soft emotions because they've already done that, way back when. Even though they may seem bulletproof, the stress will eventually begin to pull them down the *Spiral* as well).

Petersburg Revisited

It is often the case that the seasoned Combat Vet not only gets toughened to the strain of combat but also to the insane, life-threatening orders of an incompetent commander. For example, let's recall the behavior of the hard-bitten veteran infantry of Gen Birney's Corps, facing impregnable Confederate fortifications, outside of Petersburg in 1865 (as detailed in Part I). The response of these toughened Vets, when ordered to make a suicidal charge against those fortifications, was to simply remain lying prone. One of them shouted at the two regiments of enthusiastic FNGs who had also been ordered to attack: "Lie down, you damn fools, you can't take them forts!"

One regiment of FNGs did just that and survived; the other charged ahead to their deaths.

Numbed Out in Iraq

The Numbing/Toughening process is essential to survival in combat, even in modern war. Paul Rieckhoff speaks with great candor and insight as he describes his personal evolution in Iraq:

> I developed a methodical, pragmatic callousness…without (it) my men and I would have been toast. Without it, we would have stopped to dry tears instead of setting up the machine guns to eliminate the threat that could tear all our heads off with the next round.…I just stopped

caring entirely. I just went numb. Sometimes I was more than just unfeeling of their (Iraqi) pain --- I hated them for it. I hated them for giving my soldiers an opportunity to mock them and brand them an inferior culture. 'Fucking Hajis are pussies,' I'd often hear my guys say.

I'd have to admit, I thought the same thing at times. There were so many reasons for us to be angry...so many reasons to be pissed. And only one group to take it out on --- the Iraqis. (Rieckhoff 98)

Spiral I: A Shrinking Universe

Eventually, prolonged exposure to combat pushes anyone into the slipstream of this final component of Stage I. As the Numbing/Toughening component continues to impact with greater and greater force, as the debits against your physical and emotional charge account continue to accumulate, you begin to sense that your universe is shrinking.

You begin to find that the high-minded principles (political, patriotic, and religious) that motivated you at the beginning of your journey toward war now seem, most often, like distant abstractions. Sure, they still hold meaning and value in some distant way, but they have little to do with the nastiness that you have to wade through, day after day, night after night. As this process builds, your concern and investment in the world around you shrinks in uneven fits and starts, slipping into ever increasingly smaller, concentric circles.

A Combat Vet (recently returned from Iraq) described his experience of this process as follows (paraphrased):

He volunteered, driven by patriotism, a sense of duty and a desire to help the repressed Iraqi people. He also wanted to be part of the "big show," the adventure of his generation.

As the months of his deployment began to stack up, his views began to shift dramatically. He came to believe that the majority of the Iraqis "didn't give a shit"; a significant number of others he saw as fanatics whose religious beliefs gave them the right to be "vicious murders."

His view of his fellow American soldiers changed as well: from a sense of community ("we're all fighting for the right things") to a deep resentment at the disparity of experience. As is the case for most Combat Vets in most wars, he carried a special scorn toward non-combat types who had carved out for themselves "a sweet gig, way in the rear, with all the bennies and none of the sweat."

As his tour lengthened, he even began to mistrust a sister combat unit made up of "misfits and fuck ups" who "constantly got knee-deep in the shit and then expected us to bail them out."

By the end, his universe had shrunk to the point that it encompassed only the immediate circle of his most trusted comrades. He counted himself extremely lucky that he had the hard-won skills plus the good fortune to be able to carve out a safe haven of trust in that small group. Clearly, it was an exclusive, closed shop, unwelcoming to strangers until well after they had proven themselves.

His story is not unique.

Many Combat Vets from many different wars recount the same process. After WWII had ended, a Ranger staff sergeant related this story to James Jones as the two Combat Vets were working at getting drunk:

> "One day at Anzio we got eight new replacements in my platoon. We were supposed to make a little feeling attack that same day. Well, by next day, all eight of them replacements were dead, buddy. But none of the old guys were. We weren't going to send our guys out on point in a damn fool situation like that…We were sewed up tight. And we'd been together through Africa, and Sicily, and Salerno. We sent the replacements out ahead. But how am I going to explain that to my wife? She'd think it was horrible. But it was right, man, right! How are we going to send our own guys into that?" (Linderman 289)

William Manchester illustrates this phenomena as he describes the battle of wills between his own small circle of Combat Veterans, the" Raggedy Ass Marines" and an inexperienced Marine replacement

[74]

officer. They were all caught, crouching on a beach, under cover of a seawall, with Japanese machinegun fire sporadically tearing up the sand just above their heads "….when the lieutenant barked out 'Men, I know you'd like to stay here. I would myself. But those yellow bastards down the beach are killing your buddies…"

Manchester describes the stunned silence that greeted the heroic challenge from this green officer. He and his Raggedy Assed buddies had seen far too much combat to give a lot of energy to the idea of charging into the Japanese machinegun for anybody or anything.

> ….(H)e was confused. He didn't even realize that a combat man's loyalty is confined to those around him, that as far as the Raggedy Assed Marines were concerned the First Battalion might as well have belonged to a separate race. The lieutenant rose from cover; pointed at the Japanese; shouted 'Follow Me!, climbed the wall ---and was immediately stitched up and down by the bullets from a Nambu machine gun. No one else had moved. (Manchester 234-237)

To experience the process of a Shrinking Universe is a marker event for many American Combat Vets. In some ways, it is counter-intuitive to the general optimism of our national character: we tend to believe things get better with hard work and hope, not worse.

In war, this is often not the case.

(We will look at its potential long term impact on the Combat Vet in *Part III: Bringing It Home*).

The Spiral II: Combat Distress, Fatalism

Counterpoint: Small Group Loyalty

One specific aspect of the situation described just above by William Manchester is especially important as we look at emotional and spiritual survivability: "…he was confused. He didn't even realize that a combat man's loyalty is confined to those around him…."

This appears to be one of several threads of truth woven throughout the universal experience of war: soldiers immersed in combat find the strength to carry on based upon the intense loyalty that they feel to the small group to which they belong.

As they each endure the numbing/toughening process, they feel some relief knowing that their comrades are also enduring as well. Even in the face of extreme brutalization, they can hold tightly to their connection to a small, intimate group that reaffirms and protects one another, even, if necessary, at the cost of their own lives. Small units that have not bonded and have failed to develop a strong group commitment will almost always disintegrate under pressure, leaving each individual desperately trying to fend for themselves.

The following passage from *365 Days* addresses this same issue within the context of the Viet Nam War.

> No one talked. They had been out four days and they hadn't been dry once. They had taken twenty casualties in the same area, whereas just two weeks before they had taken fifteen…Strange war. Going for something they didn't believe in or for that matter didn't care about, just to make it 365 days and be done with it. They'd go though; even freaked out, they'd go…Skeptical kids who made no friends outside their own company and sometimes only in their own squads, who'd go out and tear themselves apart to help another unit and then leave when it was over without asking a name or taking a thanks, if any were offered. (Glasser 32-33)

Ripley's Dread Formula

Even with supportive counterpoints in place, continued exposure to combat inevitably draws the Veteran further down the Spiral. Some elements of that process tend to radically accelerate the speed of descent. Let's look at those elements in detail.

Amanda Ripley explores the concept of Dread extensively. She describes in great detail how Dread impacts the individual civilian when faced with potentially catastrophic situations. While her intent is to focus on the extraordinary encounter that most civilians rarely, if ever experience, her model is of great use to us in understanding the downward Spiral of combat.

Ripley has developed what she calls a "Dread formula" by integrating valuable pieces selected from an extensive review of relevant research. Her model is both straightforward and very intriguing in its simplicity. She is focusing on dread experienced by civilians in their everyday situations:

Dread = Uncontrollability + Unfamiliarity + Imaginability + Suffering + Scale of Destruction + Unfairness (Ripley 33)

So, by using this formula, we can predict that the Dread of an automobile accident would be relatively small for the average civilian. When we civilians get into a car, we assume that we have a significant degree of **Controllability** in a very **Familiar** situation. Also, we assume the potential **Scale of Destruction** and potential **Suffering** would be relatively small; **Unfairness** would not be all that important (since we assume other drivers are doing their "fair" share to make sure nothing awful happens).

In stark contrast, the case of a multi-story office building being impacted by a fuel-leaden airplane (as in 9/11) sends all of the components of the Dread formula through the roof: the individual suddenly has absolutely no control; it is a totally unexpected and unfamiliar situation, almost unimaginable (before 9/11); the suffering, the scale of destruction and the unfairness are off the charts.

So, for the average civilian, the Dread of a terrorist airplane attack is much greater than the Dread of an automobile accident. Since far more civilians will die in the latter, we can see clearly that the relative weighing of the Dread is emotionally charged, rather than rationally based.

Combat Distress

As we look at combat through the lens of the Dread formula, several very, very intriguing ideas immediately pop out at us.

For the Battlewise Combat Vet, several of the elements in the Dread formula shrink in importance while others become significantly more important.

Unfamiliarity is, of course, critical for the FNG, new to combat. But an experienced Vet has most likely passed that challenge, so not much new is going to shock him. In a similar way, the elements of **Imaginability** and **Scale of Destruction** have become less important because our Vet has most likely seen the unimaginable many times over, from the small scale to the large.

However, the other three remaining elements of Ripley's formula take us to very fertile ground as we consider the level of Distress in combat.

Part of the aura that flows from being Toughened and Battlewise is that it gives each of us the illusion that our passage through combat is <u>not totally</u> **Uncontrollable.** We can then continue to cling to the belief that, if we're smart and tough enough, we'll have some shred of control over our fate and therefore increase the chances that we can keep the Big Kahuna from landing on our heads.

Another aspect that helps keep a lid on Combat Distress is if we're fortunate enough that those around us don't experience horrible **Suffering** when they are wounded or killed. Last, but certainly not least: if our sense of **Unfairness** is kept to a minimum, then chances are that our accumulated level of Combat Distress will remain more tolerable and less incapacitating for a longer period of time.

Combat Distress: A Formula

To give us a complete tool with which we can roughly monitor Combat Distress, we need to add the element of **Exposure** to the three elements of **Uncontrollability, Suffering, and Unfairness** (identified just above).

As we've noted in numerous examples, Combat Vets who have successfully adapted to the battlefield, who have acquired the skill set necessary to survival, nonetheless begin to "wear down" as they continue to be exposed to death and mutilation. At some level each combat survivor begins to count down the number of lucky turns they have left on the roulette wheel. The more rolls of the dice that have been used up, the greater the probability the next one will really suck. Early on, each sequential brush with death was seen as a victory, proof of one's courage and competence. But eventually each new brush up against death begins to feel like a gut wrenching close call, survived only by a combination of randomness and a diminishing reserve of raw luck.

As the number of near-death Exposures continue to pile up, we become increasingly emotionally and spiritually vulnerable to that next one. By monitoring the combination these variables, we have a formula that gives us a handle on the level of stress:

Combat Distress = Exposure + Uncontrollability + Suffering + Unfairness

As the downside costs for each of these four elements continues to accumulate, our negative sum total will eventually hit a critical mass. At that point our sense of Combat Distress will mushroom into a destructive, crushing, unmanageable burden.

Any combination of these variables will do the trick. If we get caught in a situation that:

- completely destroys our cherished belief that we have some shred of control;
- if a comrade(s) suffers horribly in the process of being wounded or dying;
- if any shred of hope for a fair outcome is destroyed when a decent, beloved comrade is slaughtered/killed/maimed;
- if we simply stay in the game too long, increasing the total number of exposures until it reaches a 'straw-on-a-camels-back' amount, then the wheels can come off in a heartbeat.

A critical combination of these variables will cause our sense of Combat Distress to become overwhelming, creating a fertile landscape for the emergence of the next destructive player in this process: Fatalism.

Fatalism

Fatalism can take many forms. Some Vets describe it as simple resignation: "I have no control over any of this. Doesn't matter what I do. If I'm going to die, I'm going to die. Just screw it."

Over time, the sense that your fate is not in your hands grows ever more ominous. Paul Rieckhoff describes this process perfectly as his combat tour in Iraq grinds along, month after dusty month:

> We realize that our lives are often spared or taken by the smallest of events. Our lives become a game of inches. And soldiers count those inches often. We save them up and wonder how many more we have. We laugh about them, we trade them. We love them and hate them....It makes you feel like you have some kind of control over whether or not you die, when you know you really don't. (Rieckhoff 240)

Some soldiers resign themselves to the idea that there is a bullet or a shell out there with their name on it: "...there ain't jack shit you can do about it, so just get over it. Numb your ass out and do what you gotta do..."

First Sergeant Lipton of the *Band of Brothers* described it this way:

> "When men are in combat, the inevitability of it takes over. They are there. There is nothing they can do to change that, so they accept it. They immediately become calloused to the smell of death, the bodies, the destruction, the killing, the danger. Enemy bodies and wounded don't affect them....Their own wounded and the bodies of their friends make only a brief impression...."(Ambrose, Citizen 272)

Most Vets caught in this tailspin of Fatalism begin to detach themselves from everyone around them, even their closest comrades (since they are doomed as well). Life becomes neither precious nor sacred. Death no longer shocks nor dismays. Killing becomes the job at hand in an almost impersonal, mechanical way. Dismembered and decaying bodies are not news; they simply come with the lay of the land.

General Omar Bradley, described by many as the "GI's General" of WWII, understood this process and addressed it with unflinching honesty:

> "The rifleman trudges into battle knowing that the odds are stacked against his survival. He fights without promise of either reward or relief. Behind every river, there's another hill…and behind that hill, another river. After weeks or months on the line only a wound can offer him the comfort of safety, shelter and a bed. Those who are left to fight, fight on, evading death, but knowing that with each day of evasion they have exhausted one more chance of survival. Sooner or later, unless victory comes, this chase must end on the litter or in the grave." (Holmes 261- 262)

Concepts of patriotism, righteousness, and holiness become abstractions, distant half-forgotten memories of a different time and space.

The isolation becomes even more profound because only those (doomed) few fellow soldiers beside you have any sense of this grey, flat world that has become a permanent home.

It is the same place of empty Fatalism described so exactly by the soldier convicted of murdering his fellow soldier in movie, *The Valley of Elah*. He explains this twisted reality to the father of his murdered comrade: "It was just his night (to die). Another night it would have been me."

When our sense of Fatalism has reached full blossom and our score on the Dread formula is peaking, we have become an accident waiting to happen.

It then becomes a matter of 'when', not 'if' we finally hit bottom. Eventually the stars will come into complete alignment,

creating a perfectly tragic mix of stressors that will combine at exactly the worse time and place.

We will then be catapulted into the last turn of the downward Spiral, through Combat Distress/Fatalism into Exhaustion.

The Spiral III: Exhaustion

Finally, inevitably, the downward Spiral leads to Exhaustion.

The first telltale sign that Exhaustion is fast approaching is the occurrence of small episodes of micro-Exhaustion. These take the form of time-limited events which begin to occur more and more frequently but in an irregular pattern.

They often have the feel of an engine that is beginning a repeating cycle of stuttering, then re-starting, running, sometimes even over-amping, then stuttering again, repeating until finally, it stalls out and dies. Most likely, the amygdala, having been triggered into an alarm status so often, contributes to the unevenness of the system's response. As the cycle gains momentum, it will eventually blossom into the kind of terminal Exhaustion that Don Malarkey described in his autobiographical reveal, quoted at the opening of Part III. Like the stuttering engine, the Combat Vet will eventually quit, totally shutting down by either imploding or exploding:

> "The first bombardment taught us better, it's dirty and painful dying for your country…We sleep and eat with death. We're done for because you can't live that way and keep anything inside you." – Paul Baumer in Lewis Milestone's film *All Quiet on the Western Front*

Even after surviving the Numbing/Toughening process; even after gathering enough experience to become Battlewise; even after forming a strong bond with a small, loyal group of fellow soldiers, every Combat Vet continues to draw down their line of survival credit as each life-threatening encounter stretches out onto what appears to be an endless treadmill.

In his autobiographical description of his tour in Iraq and its aftermath, Marine Sgt. Clint Van Winkle describes the fracturing of reality that comes with Exhaustion:

> The story goes something like that, but I can't locate its actual truth. Truth lives where that piece of my soul once did and visits me briefly in sleep --- only to disappear with waking. Gunfire, destroyed vehicles, dead Marines, and Iraq are the truth. The rest is equivocal. Everything appears to me vaguely or in fragments. I guess that's how war is: It simply happens and the pieces never fit together. The mind numbs, so you can look at the dead, kill the living. (Van Winkle 198)

As the growing level of Exhaustion makes greater and greater demands on the system, the sense of Distress/Fatalism continues to quietly accumulate like fatty deposits building within the walls of an artery. Along with that accumulation, micro-Exhaustions begin to erupt in a jerky, unpredictable, uneven pattern, not unlike episodes of chest pain that foretell a heart attack. These micro-Exhaustions sometimes take on bizarre, unexpected forms. The following are classic examples.

A Nap in No Man's Land

By the barest of margins, US Army Pfc. Richard King survived the raging, brutal combat his unit encountered as it struggled to dislodge fanatical Japanese fighters from the island of Saipan in June, 1945. The Japanese were determined to defend their island to the death since it was a critical stepping stone in the American drive to gain direct access to the Japanese homeland. King would later be awarded a Silver Star for gallantry for his actions on Saipan before he was critically wounded and medically evacuated. In a letter home to his parents, written from the safety of his hospital bed, he describes a bizarre incident that perfectly fits the pattern of a micro-Exhaustion:

> "...that started our 23 straight days on the lines.... At 7:00 we shoved off in the attack. That night was the most terrible I will ever remember. The Japs pulled a banzai attack

before we could dig in. We had taken a hill, and they forced us to withdraw to safer lines so we could bring up supplies. Before we took the hill, we had a gigantic machine gun duel, and believe it or not, I went to sleep in No Man's Land for 45 minutes. When I woke up, the duel was over and 3 Jap guns knocked out. Our destroyers were throwing plenty of lead at a ridge, directly to our front." (Carroll 301)

Falling asleep in No Man's Land, under the deafening crescendo of dueling machine guns and the constant shelling from offshore warships, is unimaginable within the context of normal human experience. It is, however, a classic example of the impact micro-Exhaustion has upon the individual submerged in the underwater hell of combat.

Off Course

Robert Mason describes another classic example of micro-exhaustion in the autobiographical account of his tour in Viet Nam, *Chickenhawk*. He had already put in nine months of combat flying as a helicopter pilot for the 1st Cavalry Division when the following incident occurred. He describes simply walking to his Huey for an ordinary, first thing in the morning, flight:

> As I followed Resler down the slope, carrying my flight bag, I veered off to the left --- nothing unusual, except I was trying to walk straight. When I leaned to the right to change course, I kept going to the left. I didn't feel dizzy, just strange. I stopped for a minute and tried it again. I felt myself being tugged off track again but was able to ignore it. When I reached the ship, the feeling had gone. I shook my head. I was coming apart. (Mason 259)

"Veering off course" while on solid ground is the first stutter in the eventual shutdown of the finely tuned engine a pilot must maintain within himself to be able to survive.

The Last Dance to Exhaustion

As the incidents of micro-Exhaustion become more frequent and the Distress/Fatalism combination grows into an almost unbearable weight, the end is near. Most Combat Vets who have experienced being hurled over the edge into full-blown Exhaustion had sensed it was coming for a long while before it finally blew. For most, there was simply no way to change the dance, to get off the merry-go-round, by finding an exit to safety/sanity.

Nonetheless, the emotional, spiritual and physical shock of going over the edge is startling in a multitude of ways. The severity of that shock frequently makes the struggle to come back very, very difficult.

For some, Exhaustion takes the form of an implosion in which they turn inward, consumed by the weight of the accumulated distress and fatigue. Sometimes they simply stop, refusing to invest one more step in the insanity that surrounds them. Others seem to collapse emotionally, walking or even running away from their comrades and the battlefield.

In stark contrast, some others explode outward into a flurry of furious activity, seeking to kill or be killed, taking insane chances as they charge into the face of death. Along the way, they sometimes wreak vengeance upon a tyrannical commander who they hold responsible for arrogant mistakes that have taken the lives of fallen comrades.

Others simply become exhausted in place. Without moving their physical bodies, they distance themselves from the horror by removing themselves spiritually and psychologically.

The View from Above

As a member of an American infantry squad, caught in the death trap of a shallow ditch during WWII, Harold Leinbaugh sensed he had reached the end. He began to remove himself in place:

"We tried to keep going but were pinned down with point-blank fire only thirty or forty feet away. The fire was constant, blasting our eardrums, spraying the lip of our hollow with sheets of mud. We couldn't get off more than one shot at a time. We were trapped; we couldn't move forward or backward. I figured that was the end. We'd had it. I was looking down from above and watching the episode unfold in slow motion. I remember feeling completely detached, but terribly sorry for the guys spread-eagled in that little muddy ditch."(Linderman 75)

The View from Above II

I catapulted over the edge into Exhaustion in much the same way. In the late afternoon of his last day in the field, one of my most trusted comrades, a platoon sergeant, died in my arms. He had been shot by an NVA who wouldn't have been there had it not been for the incompetence of another American infantry unit. During the brief firefight that took his life, I killed his killer, but it simply didn't matter. My friend and comrade had been literally a couple of hours away from his helicopter ride out, after a year in the bush. None of it mattered.

During the next 24 hours, I remember watching from above as I walked across a heavily mined knoll by myself, knowing that death was near and not caring, one way or the other. Again, I watched from above as a Vietnamese interpreter forced one NVA prisoner to shoot and kill another NVA prisoner. After the company medic put me on the last helicopter out late that afternoon, I remember thinking how easy it would be to slip out the open door to the stillness of death.

It lasted for three or four days. It finally ended when I startled awake in a hospital bed, shaking and sweating. I had been silently screaming in my sleep.

Brothers in Pieces

Lt. Buck Compton was one of the most beloved and respected officers of the *Band of Brothers*. He had jumped into Normandy as the leader of 2nd platoon, was wounded and received a Silver Star. He was again wounded in Holland, was hospitalized, before once again rejoining his brothers at Bastogne, during the Battle of the Bulge.

He had physically returned but was not totally there. One member of 2nd platoon described him as being "wound up tight". Others noticed how Compton would lapse into extended silences, staring off into the distance at nothing in particular.

Immediately after a severe German shelling, Lt. Compton crawled up out of his foxhole to discover two of his favorite, veteran sergeants, sprawled helplessly on the ground, mangled and bleeding from shrapnel. They were suffering, writhing in excruciating pain and, after everything they'd been through together, it must have seemed incomprehensively unfair.

Compton began screaming incoherently for a medic as he turned and suddenly ran toward the rear, never to return again.

His disappearance over the edge, into Exhaustion, was never questioned nor judged by those remaining in the line. There was absolutely no question in their minds as to his courage. They were clear as to the contribution he had made to their survival. At the same time, they understood the price he had paid to lead them as far as he had. To this day, his comrades continue to honor him as a beloved and trusted leader.

An Almost Murder

As we discussed the components of Combat Distress, we talked about the issue of Unfairness and how it is a very critical piece of the equation. As any war wears down, grinding to a halt, as any tour of duty nears its end, a special kind of vulnerability begins to grow in the soul of the Combat Vet.

Maj. John Cochran of the US 90th Division had already had more than his share of exposure as he led his men deeper and deeper into a defeated Germany in the last days of WWII in Europe. Veteran combatants on both sides knew the end was in sight. For the vast majority of them, survival now was a precious plum, lying almost within reach and, hopefully, growing closer with each step.

Tragically, a battalion of untested, FNG Hitler Youth lay directly in Cochran's path, having set up a makeshift roadblock just outside a small German village of no military importance. They were mere boys, indoctrinated in Nazi ideology and stupid enough to still be eager to fight. After they opened fired on the lead American unit (resulting in the senseless killing of one of Cochran's veteran soldiers), Cochran ordered that the German position to be repeatedly pounded with American artillery. Finally, after taking heavy casualties, the few surviving Germans surrendered. Cochran, in a rage, confronted a young German prisoner, just after his capture. He describes the event in his own words:

> "One youth, perhaps aged 16, put up his hands....I was very emotional over the loss of a good soldier and I grabbed the kid and took off my cartridge belt. I asked him if there were more like him in the town. He gave me a stare and said 'I'd rather die than tell you anything'. I told him to pray because he was going to die. I hit him across the face with my thick, heavy belt. I was about to strike him again when I was grabbed from behind by Chaplain Kerns. He said, 'Don't!' then led the crying child away. The Chaplain had intervened not only to save a life but to prevent me from committing a murder. Had it not been for the Chaplain, I would have." (Ambrose, Citizen 439)

The sad, brutal truth is that the moral restraint exemplified in this vignette is most often absent on the battlefield in the immediate wake of unfair, senseless, uncontrolled suffering.

Retribution

Frank was the kind of guy I want on my side in a shit-kicking contest. He had survived a tour in Vietnam as a platoon sergeant with an airborne unit that had fought through far more than its fair share of crap. After months of therapy, Frank finally decided he could trust me enough to talk about his nightmare.

Frank was ten months into his tour when the wheels came off.

Frank's unit was locked in a toe-to-toe, death struggle with elements of a NVA regiment, trapped in a triple canopy jungle hell. As night fell, Frank realized that in the day's chaos, one of his squads had been cut off and was apparently surrounded. Even though he knew help would be in place by first light, he was powerless to save his guys that night. As the darkness deepened, the firing dropped off into silence. Not long after, the jungle began to echo with the screams of the members of Frank's lost squad. They were being tortured by the NVA.

By the time of first light, silence had returned.

Within the next hour, it was the NVA who were surrounded by a sister company from Frank's battalion. Only five NVA survived long enough to be captured. They were turned over to Frank and his platoon.

"We didn't torture them…though a couple of the guys wanted to. We just shot 'em, one at a time….took our time doing it….just to let'em think about it for a long while…."

"I realize as I look back at it, I was toast before it happened. I was short. My guys in the squad were short. That shit just didn't have to happen."

"It was just those screams that took me over the edge."

Frank was quiet for a long time, studying his hands, folded in his lap.

"After it was over, I just sat down under a tree and didn't move. My CO took me out of the field that afternoon. Even though he was a fuckin' lifer, he was a really good dude. He knew I was done. They could've sent me to the stockade for quittin'. Didn't much matter to me, one way or the other. I was totally fuckin' done."

Frank was quiet again.

"It was a good thing. It took a long time to begin to feel human again."

"Once you've had warm human blood sprayed all over you, it's hard to come back to life."

Thus we end *Part II: the Spiral.*

Combat Veterans

Part III: Bringing It Home

Integrating Two Worlds

In the preceding pages we have focused upon the inherent insanity of War. We have looked at the spiritual and human toll that War extracts from those who get caught in its grasp. We have looked at War's ever-increasing potential for destruction, pain and waste.

We've examined the price Combat Vets pay as they become submerged in the brutal riptide of War, losing comrades, hope and resiliency. At an extreme, we Vets can even lose our own sense of humanity. This experience marks us in ways very different than others who have not walked down that same path. Coming home, there is a strange, often times unexpected cost that we have to pay for our differentness.

Stranger in a Strange Land

For many Combat Vets, the long-awaited arrival home can have surprising, jarring twists and turns. Some of these shocks seem to come out of nowhere. They often spring up totally without warning. They are reminders, over and again, that the residue of War will reverberate within us for many years, if not forever.

In some instances these situations take on a comical tone. William Manchester's description of watching John Wayne in *The Sands of Iwo Jima* with another ex-Marine buddy is priceless (Linderman 315). They were finally asked to leave the theater because they were laughing so hard. At other times, these unexpected twists are much more binding and bruising, even alienating. Sometimes we are left feeling like we are the only person in the room with any real sense of how the world really works (more below).

Sometimes it seems the only people who can really understand are fellow Vets. Sometimes that understanding is intuitive and collective without a word being spoken.

For example, during an overnight stay at the Marine base at Da Nang in 1968, I happened to catch the John Wayne epic about Viet Nam, *The Green Berets*. The setting was a makeshift tent theater (in the late afternoon) full of Combat Vets on their way to R&R. By the end of the film, the audience was nearly in riot that ended in a surreal crescendo.

The final scene of the movie features Wayne consoling a distraught Vietnamese orphan boy who has been frantically searching a gaggle of helicopters that have just returned (after a day of combat) to an unnamed base camp (located on the shores of the sea). The boy is desperate to find his lost hero, the kind-hearted, noble American soldier who (unbeknownst to the boy) has just been killed defending freedom.

As Wayne kneels next to the boy, explaining the need for sacrifice, the sun is dramatically setting behind the two of them, into the sea.

As this ought-to-break-your-heart scene played out, a slow murmur started rumbling through the audience. Every one of us knew that when we walked out of that tent, the sun wouldn't be setting over the sea. It <u>rose</u> over the South China Sea (the only sea anywhere close to Viet Nam).

Finally, one disgusted troop stood up and cursed at the screen: "Screw you, John Wayne, you phony fuck!"

An Unexpected Gift
But there are other times when it becomes apparent that we carry an unexpected gift within us: a sense of balance and clarity. At times, our experience as Combat Vets gives us a certainty and a strength that grows directly out of the extreme stress we endured and

survived. Like the Short-timer in the film *Platoon* comments about his imminent return home: "After all this crazy shit, it's gravy!"

The bottom line comes down to this: along with the pain, sorrow and loss that is an inherent legacy from our combat experience comes an awareness and understanding of the dark aspects of life. This unvarnished reality can be priceless. As Amanda Ripley articulates so clearly in her work cited above, those that get stuck in Denial and Deliberation have really poor odds of survival. In stark contrast, those of us who can recognize things as they are, not as they "ought to be," have much better odds of dealing with the next hand life drops in our lap.

William Manchester put it this way in the first chapter of *Goodbye, Darkness*:

> I was a crack shot. I had a shifty, shambling run…coupled with a good sense of direction and a better sense of ground. To this day I check emergency exits immediately after checking into a hotel, and in bars you will find me occupying a corner table, with my flanks secure. (12)

I'll be sitting right there with him.

Vets and Therapy

Check the Box

For most Combat Vets arriving home, it makes little to no sense (as they're trying to make their way out the door) to put their fate back into the hands of military bureaucrats by voluntarily admitting they have war-related emotional/psychological pain. During the Viet Nam era, the military didn't even bother to ask. Today, the check-the-box, voluntary 'Post Deployment Health Assessment' is administered but its effectiveness is limited. There are lots of reasons to suspect that the responses are less than candid:

> Most of the guys just wanted to get the hell out of there. This was the cherry on top of a year of bureaucratic jerk-jobs…We didn't need any more briefings…There was no

mental health screenings, unless you self-diagnosed by checking certain boxes…Check the box honestly, and you could stand on another line or ten, talk to another round of pogue paper pushers and be held over for a few weeks.

We pencil whipped through those forms. Some guys told the truth; others lied to keep from being held over, or to protect their civilian jobs as cops or correction officers. Documentation certifying you as emotionally unstable doesn't do a lot for your employment prospects. In the end it didn't matter. I doubt anyone even read the forms. (Rieckhoff 254)

For those Combat Vets who do eventually come to grips with the fact that getting help is: a good idea or a great idea or an absolute necessity, a whole new set of dilemmas rears its ugly head. First and foremost, finding a good fit in a therapist isn't an easy walk in the park for lots of reasons.

A complex (and often difficult) dance typically unfolds between Combat Vets and psychotherapists (psychiatrists, psychologists, shrinks, mental health professionals of all stripes). Having spent my whole professional career (25+ years) working in the world of psychotherapy, I have acquired a bird's eye-view of these patterns. Some of it isn't pretty (as some of my fellow Vets know through their personal experience). Some of it is downright ugly. For instance:

The Ambitious Ego with Her Theory

I attended a presentation by a young psychologist at a professional conference in the early 1980s. Clearly ambitious, she was pushing hard, trying to sell her brand-spanking-new, totally made-up theory that would bring her professional fame and acclaim.

Her new theory was exquisitely simple. The critical <u>difference</u> between WWII Vets and Vietnam Vets, she declared, in terms of how they experienced combat stress, could all be traced <u>directly back to the difference in child rearing practices between the generations</u>.

To her, nothing else was important.

Thus, she described WWII Vets as more "self-reliant" compared to the Vietnam Vets, who were simply more "narcissistic."

Since Vietnam Vets had been more indulged as children (according to her theory), they were more prone to "complain" about their combat experience.

From a bird's eye view you can sees how this works: most psychotherapists, faced with the complexity of the human experience, can get easily overwhelmed. So they love to grab onto a one-size-fits-all remedy: Psychoanalysis, Psychodrama, Rapid Eye Movement Desensitization, Past Life Regression, Multiple Personality Analysis, Jungian Analysis, Faith-based Mumbo-Gumbo, Behavior Modification, blah, blah, blah. It makes no difference how absurd the starting point, if it's your precious tool, then you use it.

Young Ms. PhD, saw herself as an expert in 'Childhood Development.' So, that was the only tool she needed to carve out her theory. (My friend, Mike, commented, after reading this section: "To a person with only a hammer, the whole world looks like a nail.")

She believed she could compare and contrast the experience of WWII Vets vs. Viet Nam Vets without worrying herself with any other bothersome consideration that might muddy up her pet theory. She, in her own sense of self-importance, didn't feel any need to educate herself or to try to understand any other part of these two very complex, somewhat similar, yet extremely different worlds (WWII vs. Viet Nam).

Like it was said above, hammers and nails.

I remember listening with disbelief as she talked on and on. Without a hint of uncertainty, she had reduced an incredibly complex matrix into a simple formula. Clearly, her theoretical construction was being driven solely by her need to make a professional name for herself.

Fortunately, my great friend, Scott (a PhD psychologist himself and a former Huey door gunner) was sitting across the aisle from me. He slowly shook his head, side to side. He caught my eye, and then nodded his head toward the door:

"Buy you a beer, buddy?"

We left, laughing to ourselves, wishing her good luck.

See No Violence, Do No Violence

In another instance several years later, I was co-facilitating a support group for psychotherapists that met on a monthly basis. The purpose of the group was to discuss and brain-storm difficult cases that the group members were dealing with in their psychotherapy practices. It was a select, invitation-only group of decent, competent, experienced professionals. The group meetings were a good combination of focused work and thoughtful self-examination.

Then things got heavy. Sequentially, over a three-month period, one female member brought in a series of increasingly alarming reports:

a) At our October meeting, she talked about a worrisome case: a wealthy, charming, hard-charging, poly-drug abusing male client had gone from flirting with her, to verbally threatening her when the couples therapy she was providing he and his wife took a direction that enraged him;

b) At the next monthly meeting in November, she reported that this now-former client seemed to be stalking her at her office and making increasingly intrusive telephone calls to her home;

c) By the third month (December) someone was prowling around the outside of her remote country home on Christmas Eve, apparently searching for an unlocked window. She huddled inside, terrified, hoping that the sheriff's deputies would arrive before he broke in. They did, but he had disappeared into the fog and snow.

After she finished relating this last episode, the group fell into a tense silence (highly unusual for this group of talkers). Finally, after a long spell, I broke the silence. I asked her very quietly if she owned a gun.

"I don't believe in guns!" she snapped at me, turning away with a disdainful look on her face. I wasn't particularly surprised by her response (she later apologized to me, as she came to realize how absurd and disrespectful her knee-jerk reaction had been).

What did surprise me, however, was the group discussion that grew out of her comment. Of the fifteen practicing psychotherapists in the group, only two declared that they felt that they would be able to resort to violence in order to protect themselves ---even if they were trapped in a potentially life-threatening situation.

Consider that for a minute.

Then consider why it might be hard for a Combat Vet to make a good connection with a psychotherapist with that kind of mindset.

Of the remaining twelve, several who were mothers were clear that they would be able to use violence to protect their children (even though they felt like they wouldn't be able to do the same for themselves). The majority of the group directly acknowledged that they had never in their lives encountered a situation that might require violent self-protection. One of them even had the decency to make fun of her self-deluding innocence: "I know I've been in a protected bubble...and I'd really like to keep it that way."

Take-away:

If your psychotherapist appears to be disconnected from the reality of your experience in combat, ask them some very direct questions. Ask them about their personal beliefs about violence and self-protection; about killing and about war. Do it before you get too far into the process with them and certainly before getting too deep into the details of your experience as a Combat Vet.

Some important questions to ask:

- Do they see themselves as being capable of using violence to protect a loved one?
- Do they think they are capable of killing another human if circumstances put them in a situation where they had little or no choice?
- Can they imagine a human body torn apart?

Judith Herman, a psychiatrist and a remarkable researcher (whose work we will examine in detail below), states clearly that **Combat Veterans have a right** to expect that anyone who holds themselves out as a potential therapist has the strength and clarity to hang in there with you, no matter how ugly, violent or dark the content:

Combat veterans will not form a trusting relationship until they are convinced that the therapist can bear to hear the details of the war story. Rape survivors, hostages, political prisoners, battered women, and Holocaust survivors feel a similar mistrust of the therapist's ability to listen. In the words of one incest survivor, "These therapists sound like they have all the answers, but they back away from the real shitty stuff." (Herman 138)

Bringing It Home: A Tool Kit

In the sections that follow, we will take a close look at three overlapping areas that are tremendously important aspects of your coming home process. For each of these areas, we'll lay out a map that identifies critical crossroads that will need your extraordinary attention. These are the places where the reflexes that worked well for you in combat could now totally screw things up for you at home.

Again, we can turn to the words of Paul Rieckhoff to set the stage. He describes the long-awaited reunion with his "my girl" with remarkable self-awareness:

Seeing my girl for the first time in almost a year was awkward. It's not like the movies...my girl did jump on me and wrap her arms around me, but it didn't feel good. She was the most wonderful woman I had ever met, but it felt wrong....something about touching my wonder girlfriend with the blood and the Baghdad sand still on my boots felt unnatural. I wanted to keep the two worlds apart. I didn't want to contaminate my woman with my war....Too many emotions. I was so used to compartmentalizing them, deep in the back of my mind. Now they were bubbling up. Exposing weakness and leaving me vulnerable. I felt like she was trapping me. Boxing me in. Time to move on. (Rieckhoff 252)

Like the words of Don Malarkey (with which we opened Part II), Reickhoff does all Combat Vets the honor of honesty and directness by refusing to worship at the altar of the macho warrior.

He also pulls back the curtain on one of the many places that have the potential to get us stuck up to our hubs in a heartbeat. We'll carefully look at many of these potential traps and the specific tools you can deploy to avoid them.

We'll begin with Marriage, then move to Family, then conclude with the Healing process for you as an individual.

Marriage: The Alarm Reaction; Flooding; The Four Horsemen

John Gottman is one smart cookie.

They call him the "marriage doctor" for good reason and not just because he has a Ph.D. For almost three decades he has studied the life/death patterns of marriages and the interactional dance of couples at his clinic at the University of Washington in Seattle. He has built a laboratory in which couples can each be individually wired up (to monitor their physical responses like respiration, heart rate, blood velocity to the ear, skin conductance and muscle tension) before they begin to discuss "important issues" in their relationship.

Some of his findings are remarkable. Some were quite unexpected.

The Alarm Reaction

Although on the surface it seldom appears to be the case, in fact better than 90% of all men react both **more quickly and more physiologically intensely** than do women to negative, emotionally-laden couple interactions.

(Please read that sentence again)

Pretty amazing, huh?

On the surface, there may be few, if any, readable telltales, but, internally, men get 'upset' fast and hard: "Because of the adverse nature of diffuse autonomic arousal, men may attempt to avoid negative affect in close relationships because it is more physiologically punishing for them than for women." (Gottman, *Clinical Manual* 45).

It might be wise for you to throw away that 'seen-it-over-and-over-afternoon-woman-talk-show nonsense' about "men are from Mars, women are from Venus"… if you want to save your marriage. In fact, men do react, both quickly and intensely, to emotionally charged stuff even though it may not be obvious by reading their nonverbal expressions.

Take-away:

For women: if your map says men are out there on Mars, emotionally non-reactive and unavailable, chances are you will be inclined to crank up the intensity to get their attention. That's a really bad idea. We'll explore why in a second.

For men: if your map says that women are hard-wired for emotional neediness (since they're from Venus and you're not) and that you as a male should never go to an emotional place (being a Martian) then you've put both of you in a box. That is an L-shaped ambush for both you and your marriage.

Instead, the broad research base that Gottman has carefully built over the years points in a very different direction.

If **both** partners approach each other with care (a process that Gottman labels a "**soft startup**"), a dialogue is possible that can lead to real and sustainable problem- solving.

The difficult part is this: it's a challenge to find the internal strength and self-discipline to not go over the edge when you're being driven by raw emotion.

It's so much more tempting to "let her rip!" when emotions have finally reached a boiling point. It's so much more satisfying (in the short haul) to use a club instead of a laser beam to make your point. With the club, you're sure to get your licks in and that sure as hell feels good while you're doing it (kind of like doing shots on an empty stomach).

But you really need to ask yourself a simple question before you empty both barrels: are the payments down the line going to be worth it?

Sure, it feels great to land a couple of hard ones; the problem is there's always a cost, sometimes a huge, unexpected payback when you think it's all forgotten and everybody is over it.

At the opposite end of the reaction scale is the impulse not to explode, but instead, to very quietly implode. In this mode things still get processed in a black and white, simplistic fashion. These withdrawals begin to build an impenetrable concrete wall between partners. It's a wall that grows larger and thicker with each repeated offense. Left unchallenged, it will become more and more of a barrier to intimacy and caring, until one or both partners wakes up one morning, saying to themselves, "I just don't give a shit!"

Many experienced therapists have come to understand that a "soft startup" is an absolutely essential tool in dealing with the stress that occurs naturally in marriage. It is a tool that provides critical support to the long-term survivability of any decent marriage.

Flooding

The concept of flooding is more obvious but just as important to recognize.

Once things start to go bad, once negative emotional escalation begins, both partners tend to feed off and instantly react to their partner's last response. As a result, both are quickly thrown into an escalating state of agitation. This process Gottman describes as "flooding."

When we reach a state where our heart rate is over 95 beats per minute, as is most often the case in a heated exchange (even a quiet 'white' heat exchange), the lights are on but nobody is at home.

We lose our ability to think clearly.

We become emotionally hyper-reactive internally, even if we're not showing it externally.

(Does any of this sound familiar?)

As our thoughts begin to race, our ability to creatively problem-solve slips into a temporary coma. In such a state of arousal, we tend to create massive amounts of wounding heat and no light.

The process then tends to feed upon itself; as one partner verbally escalates the emotional intensity, the other is almost driven to respond in kind. Or even worse, to escalate the Texas Hold'em Dance with each turn of the screw: "Oh, yeah!?! You want to play that game? I'll see you and raise you double!!!"

This tit for tat, then raise you one, almost always drives both players further than they really want to go. Finally, you're both "All in!" and you don't have a clue how you got there so quickly.

In another variation of the marital dance, the ramped-up emotional intensity generated by one spouse is met with cold distance by the other. A "cold" response then elicits more heat from the "hot" spouse, which of course is met by an even colder escalation. The end result is that the "cold" partner leaves the exchange feeling battered and bruised, feeling like they have been attacked by a foaming-at-the-mouth lunatic. On the other hand, the "hot" partner storms away feeling totally invisible and desperately alone (even though they might be dimly aware that they just let their mouth overload their ass).

The toxicity of these varied dances is obvious if we stop and think about it. Once they have a foothold, they help open the floodgates, allowing entry into the relationship of the next four (uninvited, unintended, totally destructive) intruders. And, like a really bad, comic in-law movie, once they get inside your home, they're hard as hell to get rid of.

The Four Horsemen

After repeated failed attempts to talk things out, after one-too-many "hard startups" followed by "flooding," the relationship bruising has grown deeper and deeper. In the face of the increasing levels of pain and confusion, each spouse will try to make sense of what's happening to them as individuals and to the "us" of us as a couple.

This is the point where, if we're not extremely careful, the marriage will get carried away by the "Four Horsemen of the Apocalypse" (as Gottman calls them):

- Criticism
- Defensiveness

- Stonewalling
- Contempt

As they begin to gain a foothold into the relationship, each Horseman will create more fertile ground for all the others to flourish. The Horsemen tend to run together, each feeding and enhancing the others. Naturally, each increase in critical tone tends to trigger an increasingly defensive response. Over time defensive responses will morph into a massive stonewall of denial which almost inevitably feeds the cancer of bitter, resentful contempt.

It goes something like this:

"I get real tired of getting **criticized** by you, so here's back at you, plus 10%! And since I only get **defensive** crap back from you because you obviously think you're perfect, I'll be just as **defensive** in return since you're only interested in making this all about it being my fault!"

"Even if I'm wrong about something, I'll go-to-hell before I'll admit it because if I don't **stonewall** it, I'll never hear the end of it from you. You'll just push and pull me harder to get me to confess to all the other endless wrongs I've done to you in this marriage."

"Why should I own up to anything since we both know damn well that you **stonewalled** about that last crazy mistake you made, but you will never, ever own it! (Oh, god, what else have you lied about?)"

"Just like your crazy mother (or father)(ooh, that really hurts!) You're just a chip off the old block even though you say you hate the way she (he) is…

"The only feeling I have left for you is just **contempt,** just like you feel about me!"

Each of the four Horsemen has its own specific destructive potential, depending upon the frequency and intensity of its presence. Their collective impact, however, tends to gain momentum with time. The more their momentum grows, the more they gleefully wreak their destruction upon the relationship. Like an expanding plague, these four, knee-jerk reactions begin to feel like permanent reflexes, creeping into every tiny aspect of the marriage dance. When it really gets going, kids, in-laws, even friends can get sucked into its slipstream.

As they worm their way into most every interaction, they gain greater and greater momentum, eventually hurling the marriage toward disaster. By that time, the relationship is usually headed for the ICU, if not the morgue.

It's a challenge to clean up the mess they create, but it can be done.

Take-away:

1. Gottman's widely available book, *Why Marriages Succeed or Fail: and How You Can Make Yours Last,* is an easy read and **an incredibly helpful resource for any marriage, not only a marriage in trouble.** Applying the principles laid out in this book is like doing preventative maintenance on your relationship, before there's trouble. It's not much different than getting an oil change, before your engine blows up.

2. It is probably true that the "fast and hard" internal physical arousal we discussed above is even faster and harder **among all Combat Veterans, both male and female.** Those freshly back from a deployment are no doubt most vulnerable to over-reaction. While there appears to be no current research published about this subject, anecdotal reports from many different sources point in that direction. It would certainly make sense, assuming that Combat Vets especially carry within them the instantaneous combat Decision reflex we discussed above.

Let's review and summarize this extremely important concept:

If we have become attuned by our survival reflex (learned in combat) to be instantaneously reactive to a perceived threat, even at a subconscious level (remember the amygdala?), **it is reasonable to expect a similar, instantaneous reaction to anything that comes across (right or wrong) as a destructive emotional threat.**

If this assumption is true, returning Combat Vets are set up for failure if they have no understanding nor warning about this trap into which they so easily can step.

The intensity and instantaneous edginess of their reactions will be perceived by Loved Ones as way-over-the-top, disproportionate, out of whack, perhaps even assaultive.

As a consequence, some Loved Ones on the receiving end of this intensity will very quickly pull way back for their own emotional self-protection. More often than not, the Vet will sense this new pullback. This, of course, will then confirm for the Vet one of their worst fears: something is wrong but the source of the disconnection is outside of awareness.

Does this make sense?

If not, stop here and go back over the last four paragraphs. This stuff is an ounce of prevention that can save 10 metric tons of cure.

The natural reflex, the price we will pay, if we don't recognize what's going on?

Most of us would become more guarded, reactive, and distant.

A self-fulfilling downward spiral has now been born.

It will usually cause nothing but pain and confusion. A recurrent, underlying, unarticulated fear of loss will increase frustration, which will set the Vet up to get even more intensely focused, making things worse in the process.

On the other hand, for the returning Combat Vet **to simply be aware** of this tendency to instantaneously overreact creates the opportunity **to slow down or stop the escalation.** Doing so is an almost certain way to avoid doing structural damage to important relationships. The more time and space the Vet has to heal, the more accustomed they can become to slowing it down, instead of ramping it up. The more miscommunications can be handled without explosive, emotional intensity by anyone, the greater faith your Loved Ones will have that it all can be worked out. The more practiced you become in

[105]

slowing it down, the more success you will have in protecting and supporting your most important relationships.

Bringing It Home: Looking at Family

- **Rigid Roles**
- **Triangles**
- **Anticipating**
- **Rites of Passage**
- **Reflexive Payback**
- **Fragility of Life**
- **Suicide**

Rigid Roles

A military unit maintains its organizational integrity by creating and identifying a hierarchy. Specific roles are assigned to each of its members. The relative rigidity of these roles is designed to give the system strength in the face of chaos.

Yet, in the real world where the boots hit the ground, such rigidity can be a big, sometimes deadly problem. In a well-run, functional unit, roles assignments take into consideration factors like experience and personality. We looked at some classic examples in the excerpts in Part I: William Manchester, his Raggedy Asses Marines and the replacement Marine officer; Capt. John Colby and his disappearing battalion commander.

Just as it was in those combat situations, flexibility in role assignment is essential to the health and vitality of a growing family system. If one parent gets firmly stuck in the role of "the enforcer" while the other always takes the role of "the softie", the resulting lack of flexibility in the family system will allow discord to flourish. In a similar way, if one child gets stuck always being "the problem" while another is always cast as "the perfect one" or "the good kid" or "the invisible one" or "the always-loved-no-matter-what baby", trouble will inevitably follow.

As the family evolves over time, roles usually change to reflect the dynamic shifts within the system. An aging parent, for example, who is struggling with an illness, will need to relinquish their usual role of "the strong one" to other family members as the family re-organizes itself to face the new challenge.

Oftentimes the oldest child in the family of a deployed Vet will naturally assume some of the responsibilities of the absent parent. This is a natural reaction as the family struggles to adjust to the vacuum created by deployment. With the coming of the passage home, role flexibility will help everyone realign without emotional uproar or fractures that isolate family members.

In other instances, rigid role assignment has its roots buried in the distant past, outside of the awareness of all involved. Uncovering the source can be both enlightening and freeing:

A Spider Hole in Korea

Tom and Betty were nervous but determined, as they settled, side by side, onto the couch in my office for their first psychotherapy session. From their physical closeness, it was apparent that their affection for one another hadn't been dulled while surviving twenty-five years of marriage and successfully raising three kids. Betty, however, was ready "to pull her hair out" and had insisted that they seek counseling. She was clearly a no-nonsense kind of gal:

"See, I love this guy. He's a great provider who has just busted his butt providing for our family. He had to travel a lot for work, but when he was home, it was great. I used to run a pretty tight ship, so he learned to go along with the program just fine. Now the kids are all out on their own; the house is paid for, Tommy's retired and it's basically really good."

Betty's voice dropped off into hesitant silence.

"Sounds like there's a big but…" I queried.

Both Tom and Betty nodded in unison. Betty gestured to her husband: "Why don't you tell him?"

Tom shook his head 'no': "Naw, you're doing fine."

Betty shrugged, suddenly defeated. "See, that's the problem! He never speaks up. It's like I'm the 'Nag from Hell' and he's 'Mr. Nice Guy' and it's just driving me crazy!"

Betty looked at me with pleading eyes. Tom, in contrast, just shrugged again, a blank expression on his face.

I turned my focus to Tom: "Is all of this a mystery to you? I mean, clearly your wife is pretty upset but you're not as much?"

"Yeah, it upsets me that she's upset. But, I don't get what the big deal is..."

Betty clasped her head in her hands, moaning softly.

"See? I've told him a thousand times to just meet me halfway, just tell what he's thinking, instead of me all the time being the one who follows him around, trying to figure out what's going on with him and us..."

I nodded.

"Has this dance been going on for a while?"

I directed my question to them both and waited. As Betty squirmed, trying to restrain herself, Tom sat immobile, a worried look on his face. Finally, Betty couldn't wait any longer:

"Just since our youngest left. See, I always had this great give and take with the kids. They knew they could speak their minds and I'd speak mine and it'd all work out, even if we disagreed. But it doesn't work that way with Tom. He's just the great Sphinx. See what I mean?"

She gestured again at her husband and his stillness.

"So, how did you guys decide to come in and see me?"

Betty didn't even pretend to wait for Tom to respond.

"We heard from a couple of different people who had seen you in therapy. They said that you knew your stuff and that you were a Veteran."

I nodded. "That's good to hear. Those are my favorite referrals, from somebody who's been in therapy with me."

Tom was watching me closely. "So, you were in Viet Nam?" he asked.

I responded directly to him.

"Yes, '67-68, up in I Corps. I was a infantry platoon leader and company commander for a while." Tom asked several more questions about my experience, questions obviously based upon a strong base of knowledge.

"I take it that you're a Veteran, too, Tom?"

"Yeah. Korea, right at the beginning. Down around the Pusan perimeter."

"Hard times, yeah?"

He nodded. "Yeah, it was tough."

He paused, turning inward, his focus withdrawn from the social exchange. Betty glanced at me, a flurry of protective concern fluttering across her face.

"Where you stationed in Japan when the war broke out?"

Tom nodded without looking up.

"Yeah. I'd faked my birth certificate to get in the Army before anybody even knew where Korea was. Getting' in the service was the only way to get out of the hole I grew up in."

Tom took a deep breath, as he raised his focus.

"So, all of a sudden, I find myself stuck out in this little piece of hell. I'd just turned seventeen."

I nodded and waited. Tom turned back to Betty.

"I try to imagine Bobby stuck out in No Man's Land at seventeen. Hard to imagine."

Betty nodded as she took Tom's hand in hers. Tom turned back to me as he covered his wife's hand in both of his. As he spoke, Betty glanced at me again, tears shimmering in her eyes: "Bobby's our boy, our oldest. A good kid."

Tom shrugged, catching himself.

"Or, maybe I should say, a fine young man."

Betty and Tom quietly celebrated their baby together for a long moment. I waited, then, until the moment had passed, before addressing Tom: "Was it as bad as they say, before the Inchon end run?"

Tom nodded.

"Yes, even worse."

"Any particular memories stick out for you?"

He pondered, taking his time before he responded.

"Yeah. We got over run one night. Seemed like the whole North Korean army was swarming up our hill." Again, his focus turned inward. "Fortunately, or not, they'd sent me out to a spider hole, to be a listening post, in case there was a sneak attack."

He paused again, before raising his gaze.

"Didn't have to worry about that. They came screaming up that hill, bugles blazing, like all hell itself."

"So, you made it back to your lines?"

"Not a chance. I just crawled down into the bottom of that hole and didn't move a muscle the rest of the night. Lucky for me, a dead Korean soldier fell part way into the hole. Kinda covered me up, so I could stay hidden."

As we talked further, Tom became more and more relaxed. Betty listened quietly, only commenting later: "I've never heard you talk about Korean before."

Tom shrugged. "Never saw much point in talking about it, I guess."

We turned back to the problem at hand, the imbalance between Betty and Tom. Just before our session ended, I had asked Betty to stand up on a chair, one hand on her hip, shaking her other hand, with a pointed finger, down at Tom, who was huddled on the floor, his arms wrapped protectively over his head, trying to avoid the stream of demands from his wife.

They both laughed together as their dance was gently exaggerated. I asked Betty how she felt, up there in that commanding position.

"I don't like it. But, I guess that's what I do. Think I better change it." She smiled, nodding to herself.

"How would that work for you, Tom?"

He tentatively glanced up at Betty from his position on the floor. "That'd be great, I guess."

He nodded to Betty, and then to me.

"And how's it for you, huddled down there on the floor?" I asked Tom quietly. Betty's arm dropped down to her side, as Tom turned inward once again.

"I think I'm still in that spider hole…"

He didn't move as he began to weep. Betty jumped down off her chair and gathered her husband in her arms. We let the moments slowly pass.

Triangles

Triangles naturally occur in any family or system. They arise spontaneously and often simply grow out of shared styles, interests and focus. As I type these words, my wife and daughter are away, decorating my daughter's room in the house she will live in during her sophomore year in college. Their shared closeness in this process is healthy for them and our family, even though I am 'triangulated' out. It is a triangle based upon affirmation and support, not conflict.

Triangles organized around sharing and affirmation are always present in healthy, flexible family systems.

In stark contrast to healthy triangles, negative triangles organized around conflict are dangerous, even potentially disastrous to the family.

When the family begins to subdivide itself based upon members A+B forging an alliance **against** member C, conflict and resentment will inevitably follow. Each side of the triangle may include multiple members and the alliances may not be directly acknowledged nor talked about, but they are incredibly potent nonetheless. They are tell-tales that point to a system locked in a destructive dance that usually only gets worse.

Negative triangles are also usually very expensive to the individuals involved. By their very nature, a negative triangle dictates that members A+ B spend most of their interactive energy focused on what they think is wrong with C. In the process they lose the opportunity to have a celebratory, mutually affirming focus on what is positive about them and their relationship.

A returning Veteran would be wise to consider how the family and significant others have evolved in their absence.

- Are there affirming, mutually supporting triangles that have spontaneously grown in value and importance during my time away?

- How can I, as the returning Vet, fit into those triangles without disrupting them?
- How can we build other triangles with individuals or subsets of the system that meet our needs and the needs of others?
- If I return to discover my spouse and my children have grown so close that they don't seem to need me, how am I to respond?
- Will I feel even more like a "Stranger in a Strange Land"? Will I feel betrayed, deceived, "rode-hard-and-put-up-wet"?
- Will I withdraw or isolate, maybe lose myself in the numbing vacuum of an addiction, such as a series of affairs, substance abuse, and online pornography?
- If I return to find negative triangles flourishing, how can I avoid initiating or buying into even more triangles that are based on conflict or resentment? How can I help turn the system around, to help create triangles based on affirmations?
- How can we align ourselves in a way that keeps every family member out of the black and white, rigid role of the "bad one"?

These are the questions that must be asked to make re-integration healthy and sustainable with a minimum of conflict.

Fortunately for his marriage and his family, my old friend, Lieutenant Colonel John Dorf, asked himself many of these same questions upon his return from his first tour with the Special Forces in Viet Nam:

> I knew when I left that I could trust my wife to take care of things in general, especially the girls. But, come to find out when I get home, she's got things lined out just right. I found out pretty quick that I had better be careful not to mess things up. Not too easy to do, since I was so used to being the OIC (Officer in Charge). But, thankfully, I didn't get my head too buried in a dark place and we worked out a good balance.

Sure was tempting though, to try and grab those reins from her. That would've been most certainly a bad, bad idea. (Dorf, Personal communication, 2010)

Anticipating

During their deployment into combat, Veterans oftentimes get stuck "being on guard" for endless hours, days, weeks or even years; like constantly watching for and anticipating the next L-shaped ambush or for the next roadside IED. Those of us who have been stuck there know how carrying around this almost constant sense of dreadful anticipation becomes a dark, isolating, costly and mostly thankless job. As we noted in our discussion about the Spiral, being aware of your surroundings and anticipating potential danger is a critically important component of survival in combat. And indeed, there are moments in the civilian world where that reflex is a potential life-saver (like being prepared to deal with the deranged gunman in the French class at Virginia Tech; unlike the passivity of the students who continued to be shot and killed until the gunman finally took himself out).

But on the flip side of that coin, there's a terribly high price to be paid for always having your guard up. For each individual Vet, the effort required to maintain a heightened sense of guardedness can be very costly physically, emotionally, spiritually and interpersonally.

By staying on guard and anticipating danger, we keep our RPMs up way too long and way too frequently. The increased physiological stress wears away at all of our body systems, aging us and draining our resiliency. It also makes us more prone to illnesses of all stripes. It increases the likelihood that we will seek out some substance (prescription meds, alcohol, drugs, whatever) to help break the cycle, so we can simply chill out to normal. If that substance becomes the primary way we find relief, we're probably set up to climb aboard the one-way, substance abuse train to destruction.

The emotional cost of being constantly on guard is like being stuck on a thankless journey that will most likely end in isolation. Over time, we will begin to feel increasingly discounted and invisible. One of the problems with always looking for danger is that it increases the odds that we'll find it. And spiritually speaking, it's a hell of a way to inadvertently by-pass a lot of joy and light.

Finally, with our loved ones, it seems almost impossible to avoid getting forever stuck in that "up-tight, where's all the fun, life-is-a-bitch-then-you-die, Dr. Gloom and Doom" box. No matter how right you are in the long run ("I told you that kid was too young to drive!"), staying stuck and isolated in that role will drive a wedge between you and those you love, **especially** if they unite in resistance to what they see as your hyper-focus on the anticipation of danger/doom.

Rites-of-Passage

If we were able to observe a collection of family systems as they evolve over the course of the years, we would soon notice a common pattern that manifests in them all. At the points of change, where the family needs to naturally shift in its composition and purpose, flexibility becomes critically important. Most of those change points are tied to the parenting process.

Some important ones are:
- dealing with the oldest child starting school
- entering adolescence
- gaining an increased sense of self-reliance through driving, peer connection, dating
- leaving home.

For parents to guide their family through these change points in a healthy way requires that they recognize and support the subtle, but critical transformations that make these rites of passage possible.

To do so, parents need to become a tag-team, helping each other avoid painting themselves into a corner and then getting stuck. They need to help each other to let go in a healthy way, without prematurely releasing parental control. They need to help one another celebrate their child-adolescent-young adult's successes and remain available to support and help their child even when they fall flat on their face.

It is clear from our discussion of the concepts outlined in the preceding sections that there are many, many ways to get stuck.

Take-away:

Returning Vets have missed important steps in the natural evolution of their family. The opportunity to share in the process with their spouse and children is lost forever. As a result, some Vets in that situation are inclined to try to hold back the river. The illusion is that by keeping things the same for as long as possible, it seems to put on hold the next set of changes, so as to regain some of what has been lost. Others in the same situation react in the opposite direction, by distancing themselves, since they feel like the odd-person-out and it's all already slipped away from them.

For any of us, it's not a giant leap to totally withdraw if we don't feel needed to begin with.

Clearly, neither response at the opposite ends of the spectrum will work very well.

Instead, we must grab the opportunity to work with our co-parent to embrace and celebrate the change. That often demands role flexibility; supportive, affirming triangles; a relaxing of the guard as it is replaced by a sense of hopefulness and an expectation of success.

This is all good stuff to work on, especially for the Vets themselves. By pulling it off, everybody wins.

Reflexive Payback

A few weeks after coming back from Vietnam, I drove to Las Cruces, New Mexico, to re-unite with my old friend, Tony. He (also) had just gotten back from his tour as an infantry officer down in the Mekong Delta with the 9th Infantry Division. With our charming dates in tow, we found our way to a New Mexico State home football game, looking to revisit memories of the "normal" that preceded Nam. All was well until the home team scored a touchdown. Suddenly, Tony and I found ourselves staring at each other, face-to-face, each of us hugging the concrete floor of the aisle beneath the seats as the echo of celebratory cannon fire reverberated back and forth through the stadium.

As we lay there (for a long time it seemed), I think we both realized that the journey back was going to be more difficult than either of us had anticipated. There was no embarrassment for us in that moment, just an aching sense of sadness and loss. And a very real sense of isolation from the larger social network (we were, after all, the only two people in the whole stadium low-crawling on the concrete).

As we talked later, deep into the night, we realized that we both carried another post-Vietnam reflex within us that had the potential to be big trouble down the road. Before shipping to Nam, Tony and I had been in several situations together where we were able to walk away from some bullshit that could have evolved into violent confrontations. That ability to walk away was a quality we each respected in both ourselves and each other.

But things were different now. As we talked that night, we realized that we each had been forced to deal with life and death situations in Nam that demanded instant escalation to the place of "you don't want to go there, asshole!!" Now that we were back, reflexive payback seemed like it was almost hard-wired into our Combat Vet mindset.

It was a sobering but invaluable awareness to stumble across in the middle of a few cold beers. Once you've gone over that line as a Combat Vet, it's very tempting to return there. It's that sense of absolute clarity, that sense of power that's driven by a crystal clear self-righteousness and a total absence of fear: "You've created this situation, fool! Now I'm going to fix it, and you're not going to like it one damn bit!!"

It's a place we all had to go to at crunch time to survive in combat.

A classic example (easily accessed on the internet via YouTube) is a sequence in which a trooper videotapes two buddies, mounted on the lead vehicle of a US Army column in Iraq, having to deal with a civilian vehicle heading toward them at an extremely high rate of speed. After just a moment's hesitation, they open fire. They managed to light it up (at a safe distance), causing a <u>huge</u> secondary explosion. The hand-held camera shakes and lurches, as it catches the explosive-laden car literally evaporating along with its driver.

Their shouts of relief and self-righteousness rage made the hair on the back of my neck stand up: "Fuck you, bitches!!"

"Don't mess with us, ya stupid fuckers!!"

I understand.

I've been there, as has most all Combat Vets.

It's just what you got to do to survive.

But...

This same reflex becomes **a giant problem** <u>when you bring it home</u>.

Josh Brolin's character in the film *No Country for Old Men* is a classic example of this trap. He's a no-doubt tough guy, back from two combat tours in Vietnam. His reflexive willingness to go toe-to-toe with crazed killers (who are tracking down money stolen from a drug cartel) leads to the destruction of everything he loves.

As tantalizing and seductive as it may seem to go to that place on the impulse of the moment, it for sure will bring only pure craziness into the real, civilian world.

It's especially bad news if we to do it with those we love. Not to even mention the random civilian who's used to pushing his way to the front of the line without anybody ever calling him on it.

So it will be forever tempting to go to that place of "You sorry, stupid shit! You don't know who you're messin' with. I lost my fear way back when, and death doesn't scare me worth a hoot. So, bring it...."

The problem is, only bad stuff will follow if you react reflexively like the bad old days.

Fragility of Life

One of the most important markers that follow us after experiencing combat is the simple, shocking realization that life is much more fragile than one could ever imagine in civilian life. To witness the total and sometimes instantaneous transformation into death of a comrade is a life-changing event that no one ever forgets. For emergency medical personnel, firefighters and police officers, this isn't necessarily new stuff. But for the rest of us, it's an eye-opener.

Expect then that we returning Combat Vets will be hyper-attuned to issues concerning the safety of our loved ones. We tend to become even more attuned to those for whom we feel a heightened sense of protective responsibility (a vulnerable or sick child, a fellow adult who has endured some previous trauma).

All of that is well and good, but the potential rub comes when the Veteran's efforts to be protective and responsible are experienced (on the receiving end) as being controlling and invasive; even sometimes dismissively condescending:

"What, you don't think I'm capable of looking out for myself?"

"Why do you always treat me like I'm a helpless child?"

"Yeah, you enjoy being paranoid and miserable, and you want me to be, too, but no way! That's not me!"

In a similar vein, repeated messages to Loved Ones to be cautious and on guard can be taken, not as expressions of caring and concern, but as dark warnings that the world is a dangerous and ugly place. This makes fertile ground for triangles of alienation, wherein Loved Ones A+B cluster together protectively against what they see as the invasive darkness of the Veteran's war-based pain.

"Ok, we get it! Life sucks, then you die!"

"So, tell us, Dr. Doom, what's your forecast for today? Another massive car wreck? Maybe a killer earthquake? Some kinda' catastrophe, right?!!!"

A family left to drift like this, without purposeful realignment, is a setup in which everybody loses.

On the other hand, the simplest of changes can work wonders. For example, things change immediately if the Vet were to directly tell their Loved Ones A+B that what drives the worry is love and concern (obvious to you, the Vet; not necessarily obvious to A+B). That is a profoundly different message. It is the opposite of the expectation that they are naive or stupid or that they are due to fail. By communicating this simple shift of emphasis, everything changes.

Or, likewise, if the Loved Ones A+B were to directly thank the Vet for the concern and protectiveness (an appreciation obvious to A+B, but not to the Vet) and for A+B to directly express to the Vet their willingness to take the responsibility to monitor their own safety (which is the whole point, after all), everybody wins.

Suicide

It is truly one of the most confusing ironies of life.

After struggling for survival through the hell of combat, how could it be that a Combat Vet would ever consider suicide? Yet, the most recent US Army data for 2008 reports the highest number of suicides for any year since tracking began in 1980. Some estimates suggest that as many as 12,000 Vets attempt suicide each year, some 6,000 successfully.

There are some deep, dark currents at play here, stuff that really deserves our attention.

A standard issue 'Suicide Checklist' is a simple but fairly reliable screening device that many social work organizations use to try to get a handle on potentially suicidal clients. Let's see how you as a Combat Vet profile on this checklist:

- Is the subject familiar with weapons?
- Has the subject recently undergone any significant social or interpersonal upset?
- Has the subject been under any unusually strong pressure professionally or in their job setting?
- Does the subject report having been separated from loved ones or family for any significant amount of time in the recent past?
- Has the subject used substances to deal with being emotionally upset?
- Does the subject report a mistrust or lack of respect toward authority figures who have some control over their life?
- Does the subject seem familiar with or unafraid of death?
- Does the subject have easy access to a weapon?
- Does the subject report feeling either depressed or to be struggling with repressed anger?

- Does the subject report that they don't feel understood by others?
- Does the subject feel there are important parts of their life that they must hide and avoid discussing with others?
- Does the subject have the sense that their significant others could get along well without them?
- Has the subject recently lost a friend or significant other through unexpected or violent death?
- Have the subject's sleep patterns changed in a negative way?

It doesn't take much more than a casual glance at this list to see how most Combat Vets would respond with a "yes" to most, if not all of these questions. As we've discussed throughout these pages, several of the above questions have extraordinary meaning to Combat Vets: Does the subject feel there are important parts of their life that they must hide and avoid discussing with others; does the subject seem familiar with or unafraid of death; is the subject familiar with weapons?

There are several key issues that we must talk about directly so as to defuse a tragedy before it happens. Each of the following themes has the potential to haunt any Combat Vet, long after their return from war. Left unchallenged, they can grow like a cancer, eroding the will to live, dragging the Vet further and further back, into the orbit of death.

Failed Responsibility

Very few of us who have carried the responsibility of command into combat come out of that experience without significant scar tissue. The very nature of the beast dictates that, no matter how hard you try; no matter how determined you are to give it your best while you carry out your duties, bad shit happens. And when it inevitably does, it's almost impossible not to internalize a sense of failed responsibility. Even if the other ninety-nine times you nailed it, the one you missed can eat you alive. Sometimes it isn't a matter of missing anything at all; it's simply a matter of wrong place, wrong time and there's nothing you can or could have done about it.

What makes this process in combat so different from civilian life is that the stakes are so unbelievably high: a minor misstep, a tiny oversight, a hurried, harried command decision, an error made while exhausted, any or all of these can equal death and pain for those around you.

The endless second-guessing games that follow, that you (unwillingly) bring home with you, can drive you literally crazy: "if I had only"…or…"if only I hadn't"; so on and so on, endlessly.

The simple truth is that you never know when it's going to get you. In the following excerpt, we have the words of the Duke of Wellington to remind us of the awful price the weight of command can extract in a given moment.

At the tiny Indian village of Assaye, in September, 1803, Wellington led his army of 7000 into an attack upon a far superior enemy force of roughly 200,000. By carefully aligning his forces upon the battlefield before personally leading a violent assault upon the enemy core, he achieved a resounding victory against huge odds. Nonetheless, after the battle, the "Iron Duke" was haunted by an overwhelming sense of failure:

> The battle was nearly over…when they broke, resistance ended. Wellington spent little time congratulating the winners and then retired to sleep in a straw-filled farmyard. His dead numbered about 450; but the strain of the day gave him a nightmare in which "whenever I awakened it struck me I had lost all my friends, so many had I lost in that battle….In the morning I enquired anxiously after one and another; nor was I convinced that they were living til I saw them." (Keegan, Mask 147)

A remarkable quote from a commander of unquestioned strength and fortitude: "…nor was I convinced that they were living til I saw them." In those confused moments his sense of failed responsibility was so crippling that his internal pain overrode his ability to trust and internalize the words of trusted subordinates. His words ring true with remarkable candor and offer a critical reminder to us all.

Failed Courage

In the preceding pages, we've encountered instance after instance in which seasoned, respected Combat Vets 'hit the wall' as their reservoir of resiliency and strength gets drawn down to empty. As we listen to those precious first-hand accounts of Lt. Buck Compton running to the rear after the shelling at Bastogne; of Sgt. Don Malarkey contemplating shooting himself in the foot as act of desperation to escape combat; of WO Robert Mason struggling to simply walk in a straight line across a LZ to his waiting helicopter, we are reminded, once again, that our limits are finite and very real.

In stark contrast is the noble-sounding, recently-minted "Warrior Ethos" which states: "I will always place the mission first; I will never accept defeat; I will never quit; I will never leave a fallen comrade. (U.S. Army Warrior Ethos 2009). This is another classic Pentagon fairytale that fits very nicely with the latest fad that every American who puts on a uniform is a 'Hero.'

Anybody who's been there knows it just ain't so.

The trap herein is very subtle. If our sense of pride or shame prevents us from embracing the limits of our vulnerability, we are doomed to focus on failure, on that moment when exhaustion overwhelmed our resolve. If we buy into the brand new party line of always putting "the mission first", we will have a lot of body parts to police up. Then, once again, we will be left to dance, quite alone, in the endless game of shame/blame: "if I had only"…or…"if I hadn't"; so on and so on, endlessly.

Unchallenged, the process, like a growing cancerous tumor, will very quietly draw us back down the Spiral, into the orbit of death.

Again, let us return to Wellington and his candor. In the following passage, he speaks of one of his most trusted "ironsided" divisional commanders, General Sir Thomas Picton, who has 'hit the wall' in the days shortly before going into battle at Waterloo:

"In France, Picton came to me and said: 'My lord, I must give up. I am grown so nervous, that when there is any service to be done it works upon my mind so, that it is impossible for me to sleep at nights. I cannot possibly stand it, and I shall be forced to retire.' Poor fellow! He was killed a few days later."
(Keegan, Mask 162)

A Failed Buddy

A compact for survival can be an incredibly powerful motivator between fellow soldiers struggling to endure combat. When comrades pledge their faith to mutual survival, that pledge can often be the key difference between a steely determination to 'make it' and a desperate sense of hopeless isolation.

However, that pledge of mutual support can become a haunting liability when fate or bad luck or a simple mistake takes out one or more of the committed pledge-makers, leaving the survivor(s) in a vacuum of loss and grief.

The best way to illustrate this process is to share the following poignant, true story.

Ralph came into his first therapy session with me in a simmering rage. His granddaughter, Kathy, ("the only person in the world who gives a flyin' shit about me!"), drug him into my office, driven by her gnawing fear that her beloved 'Pappy' was getting ready to "take himself out."

Ralph struggled at first, declaring he had no interest in "getting my goddamned head shrunk!" With Kathy's calm, loving insistence, however, he began to gradually settle down. He didn't hesitate to declare that he was crystal clear that he had both a plan and a clear intent to commit suicide "when the time was right" and that nobody had the right to "get into my business about it!"

He softened considerably when Kathy talked, with tears streaming down her face, about how much she would miss her 'Pappy.' But, she added, that he was right: it was his business and his business alone. When I agreed with his granddaughter, Ralph became very quiet.

"The tricky part," I added, "is to know when the time is right. And when all your important business is taken care of."

Ralph nodded to himself. As the session wound down, Ralph thought that he supposed that it might be worth it to schedule another session alone with me, since I was a fellow Vet who "seems to know something 'bout this stuff" and I didn't seem to be "completely full of shit."

Turns out, back in 1942, Ralph had talked his best friend Bobby into volunteering on the buddy system so they could go fight "those sneaky Jap bastards" and get away from the humdrum monotony of their Kansas farming community. Their journey together ended on a moonless night, in an isolated shell hole on Okinawa. A single, random, unlucky round hit Bobby in the head, killing him instantly, splattering his brains all over the shell hole and all over Ralph.

"We were just kids, goddamn it." Ralph gasped between sobs. "I've been livin' on borrowed time ever since…."

In the ensuing 45 years, Ralph had never spoken to anyone about that night. The cancer of loss, shame and regret had eaten away at him, destroying two marriages, friendships and his ability to trust anyone, until Kathy came along. Now he found himself facing the final chapter of "taking himself out."

Thankfully, Ralph decided, on his terms, that he had already paid a high enough price for that old horror and that he really didn't need to eat his .357 magnum.

His story is a gift to us, however; a cautionary tale as to how loss and sorrow and shame can haunt us endlessly, unless we turn and face it, dragging it out into the light of day.

Does all of this mean that a returning Vet is at increased risk for suicide?

No, not necessarily. What it does mean is that the mystery of death is not as strange and distant to Combat Vets as it is to most civilians. It also reflects the reality that the returning Vet has been exposed to extremely stressful, raw slices of the most brutal aspects of life. But it doesn't mean that any of us are destined to take ourselves out.

The Authority Bully

In our discussion of Command Incompetence in Part I, we explored specific instances in which commanders left their troops to hang out and dry. Many Combat Veterans have had their struggle for survival made infinitely harder by a commander who was incompetent, arrogant, criminally ambitious or simply foolish.

Those returning Vets who had to deal with such a commander must remember to cut themselves an extra long fuse as they deal with power trippers after their passage home.

While in combat, some Vets are finally driven to the point that they get that pit of-your-stomach realization: "I will never again yield command-respect to anyone in a position of authority until they have earned it!!"

For anyone who has survived an idiot commander who is willing to spend lives with reckless abandon, it is liberating to reach that declaration of independence that billows up out of you in the first nanosecond immediately after the last absurd straw falls: "Screw this! And screw you!"

But we need to be aware that it also sets us up to over-react to anything that even smells of the same kind of betrayal.

We are then especially vulnerable to over-reaction when faced with a situation in which a heavy-handed meathead thinks that their position of authority gives them the right to be arbitrary and intrusive into our lives.

A two-tour Iraq Vet recently described to me a situation that came close to driving him over the edge:

Not long after returning stateside, he found himself being selected for an up-against-the-wall search by a power-tripping jerk at an airport security checkpoint. The Vet, in civilian clothes and of Hispanic descent, had to restrain himself during the search, as the security guard mumbled racial insults very quietly under his breath so that only he, the Vet, could hear. As he felt a slow, murderous rage building inside him, this Vet flashed back to a quick, intense firefight in Iraq. The sudden intrusion of the memory shook him into real-time consciousness.

He laughed to himself, and then wisely chose not to rise to the bait by over-reacting; instead, he treated the situation with total indifference, letting the guard stew alone in his own toxic, racist juices.

Bringing It Home: Healing

In 1992, Judith Lewis Herman, M.D. published her landmark book, *Trauma and Recovery*. It is a remarkable combination of research and writing, considered by many professionals to be among the best ever published in the field.

It is interesting and relevant to our dialogue that she began her research by considering the traumatic impact of violence upon a wide range of folks including survivors of rape, domestic abuse, political prisoners, hostages, Holocaust survivors and, last but not least, Combat Veterans.

First, let's look at the downside as it was revealed in Herman's work.

It is possible to identify specific patterns that tend to emerge spontaneously as a direct outgrowth of the traumatic events themselves. Clearly, they don't always occur for every survivor, every time. But to recognize these tendencies gives us forewarning that these reactions are normal and predictable and, **most importantly, that they are not indicators that we are going nuts.**

By examining them in detail, we can set the stage for turning them on their heads, to make them **work for us,** not against us.

A Life of their Own

Traumatic events produce profound and lasting changes in physiological arousal, emotion, cognition, and memory.... (T)he traumatized person may experience intense emotion but without clear memory of the event, or may remember everything in detail but without emotion. She may find herself in a constant state of vigilance and irritability without knowing why…traumatic symptoms have a tendency to become disconnected from their source and to take on a life of their own. (Herman 34)

To simplify and summarize, it seems we survivors are inclined to get stuck in one or the other of two alternate states. And sometimes they suddenly flip from one to the other:

a) We can remember painful events in great detail and when we talk about them, we do so without attaching much, if any, emotion to the telling.

b) We seem to not to have a clear memory of an event but tend to carry with us tons of emotions that keep us wound up, edgy, hyper-alert. Sometimes these super-contained emotions come spilling out for almost no (apparent) reason, leaving us, afterword, feeling even more crazy, edgy, and unstable.

The accuracy of this model no doubt rings true for many Combat Veterans reading this passage. Several notable scenes that have been depicted on film dramatically and accurately portray this phenomenon.

In the film *The Deer Hunter,* Christopher Walken has been hospitalized in Saigon after his escape from a POW cage. He is asked a simple question by a doctor, "What is your mother's maiden name?"

His dazed, confused response, marked by stuttering pain and shimmering tears, is a masterfully acted example of imploded emotions spilling out in a virtual torrent; on the surface of things, he appears 'crazy and edgy unstable,' in that his response is so out of whack, given the simplicity of the question.

In a similar vein, another remarkable scene occurs at the very end of the film *Redacted.* While attending a barroom celebration of his recent return from Iraq, a Combat Vet is pushed hard by his drunk, non-Vet male friends to tell them just one "real war story." Initially, he resists the request, but finally, reluctantly gives in.

As he begins to tell his "story," a strange mix of bitterness, suppressed rage and helplessness bubbles up out of him. He gradually falls apart as he stumbles through the telling of a horrible, violently scarring experience.

The extreme emotionality of his response might appear 'crazy' on the surface, especially to someone who has never been there.

The jerky, uneven, sometimes surprisingly unpredictable rhythm of our responses can be confusing, even disorienting (especially to ourselves). Unless we have some way to make sense of why we do what we do, it all feeds upon itself, creating a vicious, downward spiral of confusion, self-doubt, emotional and spiritual vulnerability.

Sometimes it begins to morph into self-loathing or into a very profound sense of shame: "...Man, I am really fucked up and I don't have a clue...but I better keep this shit hidden or they'll lock my ass up."

A Subdued Life of their Own

Many years ago I found myself caught in a personal experience with this process that was extremely painful and confusing.

Several months after returning from Vietnam, I had gotten involved in a very intimate relationship with a trusted female friend. We had grown very close in a relatively short period of time.

Over a casual cup of coffee one lazy morning, our conversation somehow drifted back to Vietnam. After I had described one particular "day from hell" in Nam, my friend became very silent. She had been listening very closely to me. She looked up at me with a profound sadness in her eyes: "You talk about all this horrible stuff in great detail but there's no emotion in your words. It's like when you talk about it, you're dead inside."

There was no criticism intended in her comment, only care and concern. But the fact that she meant no harm really didn't matter in that moment. Instead, I felt as if I had been totally blindsided.

Like someone that I trusted had just smacked me up against the side of the head with a baseball bat.

I immediately reacted (inside, not outside) with bewilderment ("Ok, so, how are you supposed to talk about this?"); with anger ("this is fuckin' great! I survived Nam, now I get to be screwed up the rest of my life!"); and finally with absolute fear ("oh, shit! I'm a total pysch case!")

Externally, I gave no hint to any of these reactions.

But, not unlike many other trauma survivors in the early stages of recovery, I quietly withdrew from the conversation.

And then, fairly quickly thereafter, I totally withdrew from the relationship, without any direct explanation. That reflexive withdrawal was painful and confusing to her as well as it was to me. But, at the time, I had such a strong compulsion to distance myself that I couldn't stop it. Only in retrospect, years later, did I come to recognize how my reaction had been driven by my own overwhelming sense of vulnerability and emotional nakedness. I simply couldn't endure it at the time. In fact, it would be many years later before I eventually came to realize what a great price I had paid for turning my back on her gift of insight and caring.

If we pause here long enough to look carefully at these reflexes, we can quickly see where they came from and how, at one point, they served us well. Only then can we consider what we want to do with them now as we transition home.

Stuffing It with the Partisans

As a young American OSS officer, serving with Partisans fighting Germans in occupied Yugoslavia during the summer of 1944, Franklin Lindsay saw the brutal face of war many times over. He survived, seemingly unscathed, to return home at war's end. The following excerpt is from what John Keegan calls Lindsay's "magnificent account of the partisan war", entitled *Beacons in the Night*. We pick up his narrative at the end of an intense Partisan battle to free the village of Ljubno of Germans:

"At the end of the day at Ljubno, as I left the center of the village, I suddenly came to an open field behind a peasant's house. Several men, some in bedraggled German uniforms and some in civilian clothes, were lined up facing a group of Partisans. Two Partisans had raised their submachine-guns and at that instant both opened fire on the Germans, who crumpled on the ground. Afterwards I pressed Commissar Borstner to tell me why these men had been executed. I didn't get a straight answer. All he said was that they had been guilty of atrocities against the Partisans...

"Two years later I was watching a movie in New York when something on the screen reminded me of those executions. I nearly passed out. Yet at the time in Ljubno I had not been particularly troubled by what I had seen. Psychological protective defenses were obviously at work within in me at the time; two years later they had disappeared." (Keegan, Book 435)

Take-away:

As we look back upon our lives in combat, it is clear that being able to remember incredibly painful events in detail (as in 'a' above) **without a lot of emotion was a necessary survival skill at the time.**

At the same instant, however, our ability to put a cap on intensely painful emotions **increased the pressure for them to come out sideways somewhere down the road** (as in 'b' above). You can count on it: eventually they must come out (as in the involuntary hand shaking experienced by the Captain in *Saving Private Ryan*).

The most important aspect of this model is this: we can't let the residual reflexes that saved us and protected us in combat become telltales that lead us to believe that we have become and will remain psych cases.

Instead, we need to consciously chip away at changing our old survival-based patterns, that feel ingrained but aren't; that served us well at one point but now are a needless burden.

We also need to recognize and deal with emotions directly before they become volcanoes.

And we need to become more than a little suspicious anytime we hear ourselves talking about awful shit in the same way and with the same tone that we talk about washing the car.

Disconnection: Small Scale/ Large Scale

For many survivors, disconnection from others, even supportive, committed others, flows directly from the wounding that took place during trauma. The situation just described illustrates one of the mechanisms of this Disconnection. Survivors often feel subtle judgment from others, even if none is intended.

It follows, then, that only someone who has walked in similar shoes could possibly understand:

> The role (the survivor) assigns to others may change suddenly; as a result of small lapses or disappointments…once again, there is no room for mistakes. Over time, as most people fail the survivor's exacting tests of trustworthiness, she tends to withdraw from relationships. The isolation of the survivor thus persists even after she is free. (Herman 93)

Disconnection: Small Scale

When I met him, Jake was an experienced and highly respected fire captain with an excellent, hand-picked crew. Only few minutes after he and his crew had begun their Sunday midnight shift, a fully loaded passenger jet crashed on takeoff from the local airport, less than two miles away from Jake's fire station. Even though their immediate response got them to the crash site within minutes, Jake and his crew were helpless in the face of the raging inferno caused by a full load of aviation fuel. All that was left for them to do as rescuers was to pull seventy charred bodies out of the smoking ruins of the plane's fuselage.

"It sucks, just dealing with crispy critters," one of Jake's firefighters mumbled into his bowl of cereal during their group debriefing twelve hours later. My therapy partner and I handed out our cards, warning the crew to go slow for the next 24 hours, telling them to call us if needed; that we would make ourselves immediately available for them if they felt they were about to lose it.

Six hours later Jake called my office on my emergency line. When we met later that afternoon, he described himself as "orbiting somewhere on the far side of Pluto."

Janice, Jake's wife, was both his best friend and the love of his life. She had been startled awake by a phone call from a concerned friend who happened to catch the multiple fire alarms that were triggered on the emergency scanner in the wake of the crash. She too had had a sleepless Sunday night, listening fearfully to the scanner, periodically checking on their three-year-old son Jamie, who was sleeping peacefully in his bed in the next room.

When Jake finally got home that following (Monday) morning, Janice was already getting ready for work. She had preemptively decided to make arrangements for Jamie to go to the babysitter's instead of staying home with his dad (as he usually did on Mondays).

This was the point that Jake found himself beginning to launch into orbit. He didn't need any "god damned babysitter!" he snarled at Janice and she could "just every once in a while check things out with me before going off half-cocked!!"

Janice, hurt, confused, bewildered and resentful, stormed off to work without a word. After another cup of coffee, Jake went back to work on his at-home job, nailing up siding on the family room addition he was building onto their house while Jamie played close by in his sandbox. The final straw fell on the camel's back when Jamie accidently tipped over a can of nine-penny nails, trying to help his daddy. After burying his framing hammer into the siding three or four times, Jake jerked himself to a stop long enough to get a grip on himself, comfort his crying son and call me.

On the micro scale, Jake's story exactly illustrates the process of Disconnection described above. At the very moment when Jake was most in need of his connection with his supportive wife and partner, a "small lapse" in the process between them resulted in a (temporary) rupture in their balance. Fortunately, Jake caught himself early on and was able to slow his own process, clean up the mess he had made and reconnect with Janice very quickly.

Disconnection: Large Scale

A recent article in *Newsweek* (June 22, 2009) written by Paul Rieckhoff, executive director and founder of Iraq and Afghanistan Veterans of America, contains the following quote:

> A fellow Iraq vet, a rising star at a top financial company, told me recently that in front of a room full of company shareholders, his boss turned to him and asked, "Have you ever killed someone?" It's the question most veterans dread most-being asked casually about what may be the darkest experience of their lives. His boss didn't mean to be insensitive; he just didn't know any better....This disconnection can have real consequences. (Rieckhoff, *Newsweek* 21).

Rieckhoff makes a very powerful argument that our society must avoid replicating the same simplistic stereotype, "the crazy veteran that the Vietnam generation spent decades fighting." His voice is strong and compelling, but in truth, he may be swimming upstream.

The vast majority of Americans have very little, if any, insight into the Spiral endured by Combat Veterans. Instead, they tend to fall back upon simplistic, reductionist formulas to which they have given very little thought. Hence, the totally obtuse questions cited above are not that all unusual. The net result, for many Combat Vets, is a profound sense of disconnection from the larger social body for which they have fought. This sense of disconnection also increases the appeal to join groups of fellow Veterans since they will understand without asking.

On this larger scale, we must consider the following observations from Herman:

> In situations of terror, people spontaneously seek their first source of comfort and protection. Wounded soldiers and raped women cry for their mothers, or for God. When this cry is not answered, the sense of basic trust is shattered.

Traumatized people felt utterly abandoned, utterly alone, cast out of the human and divine systems of care and protection that sustain life. Thereafter, a sense of alienation, of disconnection, pervades every relationship, from the most intimate familial bonds to the most abstract affiliations of community and religion. (Herman 52)

As we've discussed previously (in Part II), the relationship between the Combat Vet and their faith, both religious and institutional, can be extremely complex. For some, clearly, their experience in combat strengthens faith in one or both. For others, as Herman notes above, the experience can be shattering to the most basic tenets of faith. It is important to note that it is the perceived lack of response over time from a 'higher power' that is devastating and unsettling.

In the crucible of combat, the sudden realization that your life and the lives of those around you are deemed as expendable by the command structure above you is a reality check that Vets will never forget. The moment you realize that you've been sent out there to dangle as bait on the very end of a very skinny branch all by yourselves is the moment that you'll never again trust the elegant motto carved in stone over the temple door.

In a similar sense, to cling to a belief in a benevolent and omnipresent God after experiencing the horror of combat is a virtual impossibility for many Vets. The length of time one is exposed to the ongoing trauma seems to be the critical variable here.

Survivors of short-duration crises often report a strengthening of their faith after they are released from the trauma. This strengthening is often based upon their subjective belief that their prayers were "answered" (the proof being that they have been quickly released).

In stark contrast, however, survivors of longer-term trauma report feeling abandoned by their God and/or by the larger institution in which they had previously placed hope (their unit, their division, the Army, the USA, etc.). As a consequence, they most often report a total loss of faith. This is strikingly similar to the experience frequently reported by patients and their loved ones who struggle and suffer in their futile battle with chronic, long-term, degenerative disease:

> These profound alterations in the self and in relationships inevitably result in the questioning of basic tenets of faith. There are people with strong and secure belief systems who can endure the ordeals of imprisonment and emerge with their faith intact or strengthened. But these are the extraordinary few. The majority of people experience the bitterness of being forsaken by God. (Hermann 94)

Siegfried Sassoon, a young British officer who survived the trenches of WWI in northern France, expressed this strange twisting of faith with poetry and humor:

> "Poor Jim's shot through the lungs and is like to die;
> And Bert's gone syphilitic: you'll not find
> A chap who's served that hasn't found some change.
> And the Bishop said: 'The ways of God are strange!'" (2006)

Take-away:

The reflex to disconnect is a natural outgrowth of the extreme pain and the sense of abandonment that grows out of trauma.

For a survivor to carry that tendency forward into life after the traumatic reality has passed is costly and exhausting on both the small and the larger scale. The first step toward healing is for us to simply be aware that the urge to Disconnect is a predictable and normal reaction to trauma.

To understand that it is not a sign that you've become an emotional, psychological invalid is invaluable because it means you have a choice.

The second step is to explore and develop your own strategies to do something other than Disconnect.

Bringing It Home: The Damaged Self

The vast majority of the trauma survivors we have been discussing emerge out of the pain of their ordeal only after they have taken a series of major blows to their sense of self. Most rape survivors, for example, feel far less secure in their own sense of power and self-competence after the trauma than before. Likewise, former hostages will most often have a severely diminished sense of self-direction after being held captive than was the case before they were imprisoned.

Then, in addition, there are the seemingly endless "why me?" questions. In the worst case, these "why me?" questions are both asked and then answered internally with heavy-handed, damning responses:

"Well, I must not be as strong, tough, smart, competent, and worldly as I thought."
"Maybe I'm just a damned fool for getting myself into this."
"Maybe I'm just cursed."
"Maybe life is just a bag of shit no matter what you try to do."
"Maybe I can never let anyone see the real me."
"Maybe life has found me out to be the weak, pitiful coward that I always feared I might be."

This kind of private, secret inner dialogue creates a nasty hothouse for growing a crippling reflex of self-doubt and uncertainty. Left unchecked, it feeds a pervasive sense of helplessness or guilt. A harvest of self-foolishness and mistrust often follows close behind. For many Combat Veterans, survivor's guilt can manifest itself in spades, leaving unanswerable questions of "why me?" or "why not me?"

On top of all of that, Herman adds this important piece: the combination of the loss of a sense of meaning in life combined with the feeling of being cut off from a sense of the "human connection" has profound consequences to the Combat Vet:

> The risk of a post-traumatic disorder is highest of all when the survivor has been not merely a passive witness but also an active participant in violent death or atrocity. In the Vietnam War, soldiers became profoundly demoralized when victory in battle was an impossible objective and the standard of success became killing itself, as exemplified by the body count. Under these circumstances, it was not merely the exposure to death but rather the participation in meaningless acts of malicious destruction that rendered men most vulnerable to lasting psychological damage. In one study of Vietnam veterans, about 20 percent of the men admitted to having witnessed atrocities during their tour and another 9 percent acknowledged personally committing atrocities. Years after their return from the war, the most symptomatic men were those who had witnessed or participated in abusive violence. (Herman 54)

One of the major goals of this book has been to pull back the cultural curtain of softening gauze that the media and the military establishment have purposely draped around the world of War.

This curtain of illusion is supported by the implicit myth that War is noble, righteous, clean and honorable. You are seduced into believing that War is carried out by handsome youth in blue dress uniforms and white gloves, spinning polished rifles in perfect symmetry, arrayed along a majestic bluff or a picturesque shoreline. These images and this myth hide the ugly horror beneath from the average citizen and from the next gaggle of potential recruits lining up to fight for their country as "heroes."

It is not by accident that the US Marine Corps sends newly minted Marines, just graduated out of basic training, back into their home communities, decked out in handsome dress blue uniforms, before they're deployed into combat.

[138]

This illusion also hides another even more important truth that is critical to our discussion.

As we are submerged into the blind, intense brutality of War, from within each of us is drawn a darkness that is primal and obscene. For the vast majority of us who are Combat Vets, this darkness is absolutely situational, having never manifested before in our lives nor is it ever likely to occur again, **if we remain conscious and self-aware.**

Nonetheless, it is real and it is there, a marker event that we will never forget.

To have experienced that darkness in ourselves sets us apart. It also has the potential to profoundly and totally distort our sense of self.

Judith Herman identifies the process of reconciling with oneself as a critical component in the final stage of recovery from any and all manner of trauma. Thus, a rape survivor must both remember and draw strength from the most valuable, powerful aspects of themselves that were central to their being **before the intrusion of the trauma:**

> Gaining possession of oneself often requires repudiating those aspects of the self that were imposed by the trauma. As the survivor sheds her victim identity, she may also choose to renounce parts of herself that have felt almost intrinsic to her being. (Herman 203)

In this instance, Herman is underscoring the critical importance of freeing oneself from the sense of being a 'victim'. To heal, rape survivors must free themselves from the post-trauma tendency toward passivity that arises in the face of potential violence. They must, instead, tap into and feed any sense of strength that they held within themselves **before the trauma distorted their sense of self.**

In this way, it will be possible to rebuild a place within from which it is possible for the survivor to fight for herself and to never, ever be 'helpless' again.

Combat Veterans

In a parallel sense, Combat Veterans must remember, value and draw deeply upon the decent, humane aspects of themselves that were an important part of their being before becoming distorted and twisted by being submerged in War.

As Combat Veterans, we must remain purposeful in our determination to eliminate our combat-induced, acquired reflexes:

A) to reflexively react powerfully with violence and brutality, thereby bypassing fear.

B) to look for the dark side in others and remain ever-vigilant

C) to ignore all soft emotions for the sake of power and invulnerability

D) to view the world through a simple lens that just sees "Us vs. Them"

E) to believe that it is just a matter of time before those closest to you die or go away

F) that at the end of the journey it's truly ever person for themselves

All of the above are classic combat survival mechanisms. If we carry them forward with us during our passage home, it will be crippling to us and to those that love us.

Collectively, they have the potential to become a destructive, pain-filled legacy if we let it let go of their leash, emotionally and/or physically. If we don't fight to change that legacy, it will quickly lead to isolation and loss.

So this is our most important battle.

We must remain conscious and challenge that cultural stereotype that we carry **within us:** that we, as Combat Vets, are only a hair's breadth away from being triggered back into a spontaneous, powerful orgy of violence and mayhem.

It is critical to our healing that we remain aware that this reflexive violence is now a crippling legacy of War that, unchallenged, has the potential to curse us forever.

Left unchallenged, it will drive us to our doom like an over-burdened, weary pack animal, carrying unendurable loads of pain, violence and loss down a descending, isolated trail into darkness.

We must find the clarity and resolve to never, ever go to that place of being a 'killer' again:

> As survivors recognize and 'let go' of those aspects of themselves that were formed by the traumatic environment, they also become more forgiving of themselves. They are more willing to acknowledge the damage done to their character when they no longer feel that such damage must be permanent. (Herman 203)

Here we are in the heart of the healing process.

We will close with the words of a fellow soldier who has been there.

As a young lieutenant in Vietnam, Max Cleland lost both legs and an arm in combat. Undeterred by his crippling wounds, he would eventually win the race for the US Senate from the state of Georgia.

More than thirty years after his medical evacuation from Vietnam, Cleland returned to Walter Reed Medical Center to seek treatment for PTSD. When asked what message he would like to pass on to his fellow Veterans, this was his reply:

> "You may never get over the war in which you served, but don't give up hope. You are not alone in your suffering, and counseling can make the best of a bad situation. The scars will be there, but a freshness of life will begin to emerge." (Oct. 4, 2009)

And so it goes.

Combat Veterans

Part IV: The Nature of War

We began this journey back in **Part I: What They Didn't Tell You.**
From there, we tracked the predictable, painful downward spiral of
combat in **Part II: the Spiral,** as is experienced by most Combat
Veterans. From there, we turned to a detailed exploration into the
journey back in **Part III: Bringing It Home.**

Now we'll look at how War has transformed itself over the last
six centuries; how it takes on the qualities of a living organism,
following its own evolutionary path. How it has led us to where we are
today.

America's Endless Wars

If we were to slowly travel back through the years since the
horror of September 11, 2001, most patriotic Americans would be
flooded with many painful crosscurrents: emotional, spiritual and
psychological.

The images would stack up, one upon another, into a
monument of conflict and contrast:

- Flag-draped coffins, row upon row, filling the belly of
  Air Force cargo planes.
- A toppled statue of Hussein being beaten with shoes
- A thin-skinned Hummer being hurled into the air by
  the sudden violence of an IED
- The bridge of an aircraft carrier draped with 'Mission
  Accomplished'
- A high school gym full of National Guardsmen saying
  another tearful goodbye to their loved ones.

These images and a multitude of even more personal, private
memories would then fill in the details of our personal picture of War.

[143]

Be it the 'War on Terror' or the 'Iraq War' or the 'War in Afghanistan', the similarities would far outweigh the differences.

But...

What if that very personal process leaves out important parts of the larger picture? Parts whose absence handicaps or even distorts our individual and collective understanding of War?

It may even be that these missing parts are so subtle and so complex that only those who have the time to ponder them in great detail get a clear grasp of their dirty, big-little secrets.

If we had a chance to sit down over a cup of coffee and talk with one of those "in the know" kind of folks, what would you guess they would say? What small but desperately important little details could we gather from them that would give us a clearer picture?

Let's do and see what we find.

Bruce Catton, one of America's most widely respected 20th century historians, was one of those 'in the know' folks. He made this stunning observation while writing about the American Civil War, back in 1971:

> A singular fact about modern war is that it takes charge. Once begun it has to be carried to its conclusion and carrying it there sets in motion events that are beyond men's control. Doing what has to be done to win, men perform acts that alter the very soil in which society's roots are nourished.
> (Catton 19)

Interesting, huh? Could he have been talking about Guantanamo, about 'enhanced interrogation', about 'collateral damage', about 'force retention'?

Wait, there's more.

John Keegan, a British historian known for his integrity and insight, offers an even wider view of War as he pans further back. Writing in 1976 he seems to foretell the dilemmas with which we still struggle today, in Iraq, in Afghanistan, in the "War on Terror":

> War, in a Christian theology, is a sinful activity, unless carried on within a framework of rules which few commanders

are in practice able to obey; in particular those which demand that he shall have a just aim and a reasonable expectation of victory. Any objective study quickly reveals, however, that most wars are begun for reasons which have nothing to do with justice, have results quite different from those proclaimed as their objects, if indeed they have any clear cut result at all, and visit during their course a great deal of casual suffering on the innocent. (Keegan, Book 60)

Could he be right?

Could it be that "wars are begun for reasons that have nothing to do with justice" and that eventually, whether intended or not, they will "visit in their course a great deal of casual suffering on the innocent"?

High Purpose, Noble Goals

By simply glancing at recent history, we can identify important proclamations that mark the beginning of most modern Wars; we can compare these proclamations with the reality that mark the endings of that same war. In fact, some very interesting contrasts pop up. The following is an interesting example.

At the outbreak of World War II in September, 1939, the British government forbid British Bomber Command from sending any of proposed bombing missions over Germany because the government was very seriously concerned that potential damage to 'private property' (by errant bombs) be avoided, if at all possible.

Shortly thereafter, in August of 1941, (four months before America entered WWII) Winston Churchill and Franklin Roosevelt laid down the principles of the 'Four Freedoms' within the Atlantic Charter. Two of the principles put forth in this noble and high-minded document proclaimed: "all the nations of the world should be free from aggression' and that all peoples should enjoy "the freedom from want and fear".

Yet, by the end of WWII, every urban center in Germany with an industrial component of even the most minor importance had been reduced to smoldering rubble by the combination of American day, and British night, bombing raids. Countless numbers of civilian non-combatants---children, women and elderly---were slaughtered in the process.

What this meant was that a rising proportion of first British, and then American resources were diverted into the destruction of German and Japanese cities --- in other words, the slaughter of civilians. This was precisely the policy the US State Department had denounced as 'unwarranted and contrary to principles of law and humanity' when the Japanese had first bombed Chinese cities. It was precisely the policy that Neville Chamberlain had once dismissed as 'mere terrorism', a policy to which 'His Majesty's government [would] never resort.' (Ferguson 560)

By the time WWII finally ended, bombing techniques and weaponry had evolved in ways that were unimaginable back at the beginning of the war in 1939. A single American night-time raid on Tokyo, targeting the city's primarily wood and paper houses with incendiary bombs, created a self-feeding firestorm that killed over 100,000 civilians.

One American pilot described the sight:

"Suddenly...I saw a glow on the horizon like the sun rising or maybe the moon. The whole city of Tokyo was below us stretching from wingtip to wingtip, ablaze in one enormous fire with yet more fountains of flame pouring down from the B-29s. The black smoke billowed up thousands of feet causing powerful thermal currents that buffeted our plane severely, bringing with it the horrible smell of burning flesh." (Hastings, Retribution 297)

Curtis LeMay, the Air Force general who was the chief architect of this attack design, was pleased with the outcome. He described his policy as "Bomb and burn 'em till they quit." His boss, General Arnold, wrote the following congratulatory note to LeMay

So, we're left wondering: what happened?

How did the Allied leadership, led by Churchill and Roosevelt, travel so far from the humanistic goals pronounced in the Four Freedoms?

How did it come to pass that these young American pilots, decent and responsible kids who willingly put their lives on the line every time they flew over Japan, got caught up in this highly efficient machine of mass human slaughter?

Ernst Hemingway had a sense of foreboding, warning America of this process as early as 1942, as he wrote his introduction to his book, *Men at War:* "We must win it (WWII) never forgetting what we are fighting for, in order that while we are fighting Fascism we do not slip into the ideas and ideals of Fascism." (Hackworth 830)

Could it be that Catton and Keegan are right?

Could it be that War is a power unto itself? That once we "let loose the dogs of war" (to use Shakespeare's metaphor) we surrender our fate to an organism that quickly frees itself from human restraint, morphing and evolving as it will?

To consider that question, let's take a look at a small village in northern France in October, 1415.

The Evolution of War: Agincourt

In his engaging book, *The Face of War*, John Keegan closely examines the 'human' component of battle as it has evolved over the last six centuries, beginning with the battle of Agincourt in northern France in October of 1415.

For the French and English knights (bowman and men-at-arms) gathering in a muddy field on the outskirts of the tiny French village of Agincourt, battle was very close and personal; most often, face-to-face. At its height, the battle was brutal and intense but the slaughter was limited. Let's let John Keegan be our guide:

> The rhythm of the fighting and its duration were in consequence dictated by human limitations: a man gained ground on his opponent, scored a hit, felt his sword arm tire, knew that he must win in the next five minutes or be done for;

and *pari passu*, the same rhythms imposed themselves on his opponent. Because medieval armies were small, and battles were often fought without either side holding men in reserve, these rhythms determined the length of combat. And because the power of weapons was not very much greater than the muscle power of those who wielded them, the wounds inflicted were little different from the wounds of everyday life. (Keegan, Face 320)

By the end of the day the English emerged victorious, due in large measure to the fact that the massed English bowmen were able to slaughter the mounted French knights as they struggled slowly through the morass of a muddy, freshly plowed field. As well, a critical improvement in the design of the tip of the English arrow gave it a vastly improved penetrating power, enough to render the French armor significantly less effective. (Is this a foreshadowing of IEDs and armored personnel carriers?)

Some historians have described Agincourt as "the end of Chivalry" in that peasants, armed with a technologically enhanced weapon, could now slaughter armed knights. Let's flash forward four centuries...

The Evolution of War: Waterloo

The nature of battle had evolved in some interesting ways by the Battle of Waterloo in 1815. The gunpowder battles, as Keegan calls them, were significantly more impersonal than those of the earlier age. Soldiers were drilled to operate and fight in units, unlike the rather chaotic organization of the battlefield at Agincourt (which involved more one-on-one, face-to-face engagement). The new technology of the smooth-bore musket required that troops be drilled in the loading and firing of this, a cumbersome and largely inaccurate weapon.

Portable artillery added to the noise, smoke and confusion of the battlefield but was highly inaccurate except at very close range. The fighting was almost always limited to daylight hours, with formal structures laying out the protocol for accepting surrenders, the humane treatment of prisoners and a general concern to do no harm to non-combatants.

The valor of the individual became somewhat less distinguishable as large bodies of men collided in the swirling confusion of the battlefield. The heroic cavalry charge still held its place as the most dramatic, tide-changing event to emerge in both legend and cultural bias.

The emphasis upon individual courage and valor would remain central to the culturally-based warrior myth even yet, with dire consequences to follow.

The Evolution of War: The American Civil War

More than a few historians of merit argue that in the course of the American Civil War (1861-1865), the face of War was changed forever. The opening battles of this bloody and bitter conflict featured many of the same aspects of the 'heroic' marital spirit that was manifested at Waterloo.

Gallantly waving battle flags, units of uniformed, courageous soldiers marched in unison into battle, accompanied by the thundering pounding of proud cavalry who hurled themselves fearlessly into the melee. The generals, both North and South, had earned their spurs a decade before, during the Mexican War, a war that in many ways closely resembled Waterloo (unfortunately as it turns out): "Here, closed rank linear formation and very aggressive Napoleonic bayonet charges bore spectacular results and relative few casualties in a series of stunning American victories. It was a lesson the participants would not soon forget." (O'Connell 197)

The military leadership of both North and South had every reason to believe that the battle tactics that had worked against the Mexicans would work in this new war.

Tragically, they couldn't have been further from the truth. Despite the reality before them, they insisted upon re-fighting 'the last war' (the recurring phenomena we will discuss in detail later). In that process, they continued to ignore the fact that the standard weapon for soldiers on both sides was no longer the smooth-bore musket (a highly inaccurate weapon in the best of circumstance), but its new cousin, the next step in the evolutionary ladder: the rifled musket.

As the common soldiers on both sides became more and more efficient with this readily available, mass-produced rifled musket, their effective killing range grew to over one thousand yards. Thus, a new truth emerged on the Civil War battlefield: a well-entrenched infantry unit, supplied with adequate ammunition, would repulse and essentially destroy a numerically superior attacking force, time and time and time again: "It was not war- it was murder," concluded Gen. Daniel Hill after his division had lost two thousand of its sixty-five hundred men attacking Union positions at Malvern Hill." (O'Connell 197)

The generals, both North and South, were not interested in reality. Instead, they clung passionately, blindly to their belief in the 'attack'. Both North and South believed that the moral superiority of their cause would eventually result in the imposition of their will upon the enemy. If, they, as commanders could spur their troops on to greater and greater sacrifice, then their 'Noble Cause' would be won. O'Connell continues:

> Instead, the opposing forces found themselves locked in a bloodbath, with the aggressive Southerners, urged on by the ever–combative Jefferson Davis, suffering particularly intensely. In eight of the first twelve big battles, Confederates assumed the tactical offensive, and lost ninety-seven thousand men doing so. Altogether, the South suffered 175,000 battle casualties in the first twenty-seven months of fighting, a figure somewhat higher than the entire Confederate military establishment in 1861. (197)

Ulysses S. Grant, the Union general who took over command of the Army of the Potomac in 1864, managed to sustain sixty-four thousand casualties in less than three months of campaigning.

> Unlike their officers, foot soldiers drew an altogether more practical, if less heroic, conclusion as to the tactical

significance of new weaponry, and sought cover and defensible positions whenever possible…

And, in fact, a better indication of the true tactical situation was the spectacle of Union troops pinning their names to their uniforms shortly before the notorious frontal assault on Confederate positions at Cold Harbor on 3 June so that their corpses might be better identified after the battle. (O'Connell 198)

The Evolution of War: Patterns Emerge

As we continue to follow this evolving timeline, several patterns are revealed:

1. Advances in technology and weaponry impose themselves incessantly into the battlefield and dramatically transform the nature of the conflict.
2. Military leaders reflexively fight 'the last war' and are either unwilling or unable to deal with a new, evolving reality.

The Evolution of War: The Somme

By the beginning of WWI the evolution in military hardware was following a truly dazzling trajectory. The range and complexity of indirect fire weapons, howitzers, mortars, artillery (from horse-drawn field pieces to huge railway guns) made it possible to deliver (literally) earth-shaking death upon the distant, unseen enemy. But no single weapon transformed the WWI battlefield more than the machine gun with its ability to deal out death in a steady, easily maintained stream.

Given that all of the generals (French, English, German, Russian, it mattered not) continued to desperately cling to their faith in the 'courageous' attack, the table was set for slaughter of almost unimaginable proportions. The British assault at the Somme was but one example in this tragic pattern.

By the summer of 1916, after two frustrating years of war, the British were determined to break the stalemate in the trenches in northern France. In an intense preparatory bombardment lasting seven days, over 1,500,000 British shells pounded the German defensive trench works, both day and night. In theory, the British generals believed their troops would be able to walk, unmolested, through the multiple layers of the now-destroyed German fortifications.

As the bombardment ceased, British troops climbed out of their trenches to begin the attack; at the same moment the surviving Germans crawled out of their underground bunkers, manned their machine guns and the slaughter began.

In the ensuing attack, the British suffered over sixty thousand casualties; twenty-one thousand of those in the first few moments of the attack. The impetus of the attack died quickly as dazed, confused survivors became overwhelmed by the enormous losses all around them.

Keegan argues that the trenches of the Somme foreshadow the coming, twenty five years later, of the German concentration camps of Hitler's Third Reich:

> ...those long docile lines of young men, shoddily uniformed, heavily burdened, numbered about their necks, plodding forward across a featureless landscape to their own extermination inside the barbed wire. Accounts of the Somme produce in readers and audiences much the same range of emotions as do descriptions of the running of Auschwitz – guilty fascination, incredulity, horror, disgust, pity and anger. (Keegan, Face 255)

A Power unto Itself

We have explored the nature of War over the centuries and identified patterns that clearly point to a singular truth: War, by its very nature, is a power unto itself.

Let us give the final word to Winston Churchill, a participant in and witness of many wars:

> Never, never, never believe any war will be smooth and easy, or that anyone who embarks on the strange voyage

can measure the tides and hurricanes he will encounter. The statesman who yields to war fever must realize that once the signal is given, he is no longer the master of policy but the slave of unforeseeable and uncontrollable events. (Hastings, Armageddon 475)

Combat Veterans

Bibliography

Ambrose, Stephen E. *Americans at War*. Jackson: University of
Mississippi, 1997. Print.

Ambrose, Stephen E. *Band of Brothers*. New York: Simon & Schuster,
1996. Print.

Ambrose, Stephen E. *Citizen Soldiers*. New York: Simon & Schuster,
1997. Print.

Catton, Bruce. *A Stillness at Appomattox*. New York: Doubleday,
1953. Print.

Cowley, Robert, ed. *No End Save Victory*. New York: G.P. Putman's
Sons, 2001. Print.

Davis, Burke. *Gray Fox*. New York: Wings, 1956. Print.

D'Este, Carlo. *Patton, a Genius for War*. New York: Harper Collins,
1995. Print.

Dower, John W. *War Without Mercy*. New York: Pantheon, 1986.
Print.

Ferguson, Niall. *The War of the World: Twentieth-century Conflict and
the Descent of the West*. New York: Penguin, 2006. Print.

Foote, Shelby. *The Civil War: A Narrative, Fort Sumter to Perryville*.
New York: Random House, 1958. Print.

Fussell, Paul. *Thank god for the atom bomb, and other essays*. New
York: Ballantine, 1990. Print.

Fussell, Paul. *Wartime*. New York: Oxford UP, 1989. Print.

Glasser, Ronald J. *365 Days*. New York: George Braziller, 1971. Print.

Gottman, John. *Why Marriages Succeed or Fail*. Fireside, 1994. Print.

Hackworth, David H., and Julie Sherman. *About Face*. New York:
Simon & Schuster, 1989. Print.

Hastings, Max. *Armageddon*. New York: Alfred A. Knopf, 2004. Print.

Hastings, Max. *Retribution*. New York: Alfred A. Knopf, 2007. Print.

Hastings, Max. *The Korean War*. New York: Simon & Schuster, 1987.
Print.

Herman, Judith L. *Trauma and Recovery*. Basic, 1992. Print.

Holmes, Richard. *Acts of War: the Behavior of Men in Battle*. New York: Free, 1986. Print.

Keegan, John, ed. *The Book of War*. New York: Viking, 1999. Print.

Keegan, John. *The Face of Battle*. New York: Barnes & Noble, 1993. Print.

Keegan, John. *The Mask of Command*. New York: Penguin, 1987. Print.

Keegan, John. *The Price of Admiralty*. New York: Viking, 1988. Print.

Krakauer, Jon. *Where Men Win Glory*. New York: Doubleday, 2009. Print.

Lawrence, T. E. *Seven Pillars of Wisdom: a Triumph*. New York: Anchor, 1991. Print.

LeDoux, Joseph. *The Emotional Brain*. New York: Simon & Schuster, 1996. Print.

Linderman, Gerald F. *The World Within War*. New York: Free, 1997. Print.

Lindsay, Franklin. *Beacons in the Night*. Palo Alto: Stanford, 1993. Print.

Lindy, Jacob D. *Vietnam: A Casebook*. New York: Brunner/Mazel, 1988. Print.

Malarkey, Don, and Bob Welch. *Easy Company Soldier: the Legendary Battles of a Sergeant from World War II's "Band of Brothers"* New York: St. Martin's, 2008. Print.

Manchester, William Raymond. *Goodbye, Darkness: a Memoir of the Pacific War*. Boston: Little, Brown, 1980. Print.

Mason, Robert. *Chickenhawk*. New York: Viking, 1983. Print.

O'Connell, Robert L. *Of Arms and Men*. New York: Oxford UP, 1989. Print.

Rieckhoff, Paul. *Chasing Ghosts: a Soldier's Fight for America from Baghdad to Washington*. New York: NAL Caliber, 2006. Print.

Ripley, Amanda. *The Unthinkable: Who Survives When Disaster Strikes and Why*. New York: Crown, 2008. Print.

Severo, Richard, and Lewis Milford. *The Wages of War*. New York: Simon & Schuster, 1989. Print.

Van Winkle, Clint. *Soft Spots: a Marine's Memoir of Combat and Post-traumatic Stress Disorder*. New York: St. Martin's, 2009. Print.

Film Cited

The Deer Hunter. Dir. Michael Cimino. Perf. Robert DeNiro, Christopher Waken. Universal Pictures, 1978. Film.

In the Valley of Elah. Dir. Paul Haggis. Perf. Tommy Lee Jones, Charlize Theron. Warner Independent Pictures, 2007. Film.

Lawrence of Arabia. Dir. David Lean. Perf. Peter O'Toole, Omar Shariff. Columbia Pictures, 1962. Film.

No Country For Old Men. Dir. Joel Coen and Ethan Coen. Perf. Josh Brolin, Javier Barden. Miramex Films, 2007. Film.

Platoon. Dir. Oliver Stone. Perf. Charlie Sheen, Tom Berenger. Metro Goldwyn Mayer, 1986. Film.

Redacted. Dir. Brian DePalma. Perf. Kel O'Neill, Daniel Steward Sherman. Magnolia Pictures, 2007. Film.

Saving Private Ryan. Dir. Steven Spielberg. Perf. Tom Hanks, Tom Sizemore. Dream Works, 1998. Film.

DVD Cited

All Quiet on the Western Front. Dir. Delbert Mann. Perf. Richard Thomas, Ernest Borgnine. 2001. DVD.

Band of Brothers. Dir. Phillip A. Robinson, et al. Perf. Damian Lewis, Ron Livingston. 2001. DVD.

Magazine Cited

Boal, Mark. "Death and Dishonor*" Playboy* May, 2004

Orr, J. Scott. "Helping Soldiers Heal.*" Parade* Oct.4, 2009: 6

Rieckhoff, Paul. "Who Are You Calling Rambo?" *Newsweek* June 22, 2009: 21

Combat Veterans

About the Author

Bill DeWitt, MA, MFT, LDAC served as an infantry platoon leader and company commander in Viet Nam, 1967-68.

His 25+ year career in counseling began in a "street program" for substance abusing adolescents. After obtaining his Masters in Counseling, DeWitt became a Licensed Drug and Alcohol Counselor as well as nationally licensed Marriage and Family Therapist.

His career path has included: counseling at a maximum security prison and woman's prison; Family Therapy consulting for a female adolescent residential drug treatment program; an external consultant for First Responders (fire, police, EMTs) in crisis; staff Consultant for an AIDS/HIV clinic.

Through a National Institute of Mental Health grant project, he was instrumental in developing a Family Therapy training package that could be delivered to community-based counselors. He trained that package in a wide variety of setting throughout the western states and to Armed Forces Counselors in the Pacific basin. He has presented at national conferences and to professional organizations.

Throughout his career, DeWitt has had the opportunity to work with Combat Veterans (and their families) from every war, WWII to Iraq/Afghanistan.

He currently lives in Oregon with his wife and daughter. He can be reached at *Bill@combatveterans-bringingithome.com.*

5006567R0

Made in the USA
Charleston, SC
16 April 2010